Immunomodulatory Effects of Nanomaterials

Woodhead Publishing Series in Biomaterials

Immunomodulatory Effects of Nanomaterials

Assessment and Analysis

Edited by

MAHMOUD ELSABAHY

School of Biotechnology, Badr University in Cairo, Badr City, Cairo, Egypt

ELSEVIER

WP WOODHEAD PUBLISHING

An imprint of Elsevier

Woodhead Publishing is an imprint of Elsevier
50 Hampshire Street, 5th Floor, Cambridge, MA 02139, United States
The Boulevard, Langford Lane, Kidlington, OX5 1GB, United Kingdom

ISBN: 978-0-323-90604-3 (print)

ISBN: 978-0-323-90824-5 (online)

Publisher: Matthew Deans
Acquisitions Editor: Sabrina Webber
Editorial Project Manager: Rafael G. Trombaco
Production Project Manager: Nirmala Arumugam
Cover Designer: Vicky Pearson Esser

Typeset by MPS Limited, Chennai, India

Contents

List of contributors

Omar A. Abdelaziz
Nanomedicine Laboratory, Center for Materials Science, Zewail City of Science and Technology, Giza, Egypt

Ahmed S. Abo Dena
Nanomedicine Laboratory, Center for Materials Science, Zewail City of Science and Technology, Giza, Egypt; Pharmaceutical Chemistry Department, National Organization for Drug Control and Research (NODCAR), Giza, Egypt

Noura G. Eissa
Department of Pharmaceutics and Industrial Pharmacy, Faculty of Pharmacy, Zagazig University, Zagazig, Egypt

Mahmoud Elsabahy
School of Biotechnology and Science Academy, Badr University in Cairo, Badr City, Cairo, Egypt; Department of Chemistry, Laboratory for Synthetic-Biologic Interactions, Texas A&M University, College Station, TX, United States; Misr University for Science and Technology, 6th of October City, Giza, Egypt; Department of Pharmaceutics, Faculty of Pharmacy, Assiut University, Assiut, Egypt

Ibrahim M. El-Sherbiny
Nanomedicine Laboratory, Center for Materials Science, Zewail City of Science and Technology, Giza, Egypt

Gamal Esmat
Badr University in Cairo, Badr City, Cairo, Egypt; Department of Hepatogastroenterology and Infectious Diseases, Faculty of Medicine, Cairo University, Cairo, Egypt

Ashraf H. Ghaleb
Misr University for Science and Technology, 6th of October City, Giza, Egypt; Department of Surgery, Faculty of Medicine, Cairo University, Cairo, Egypt

Mostafa A. Hamad
Department of Surgery, Faculty of Medicine, Assiut University, Assiut, Egypt

Nourhan Mohamed
Department of Microbiology and Immunology, Faculty of Pharmacy, Sphinx University, Assiut, Egypt

Paul W. Rhyne
Bill & Melinda Gates Medical Research Institute, Cambridge, MA, United States

Karen L. Wooley
Department of Chemistry, Laboratory for Synthetic-Biologic Interactions, Texas A&M University, College Station, TX, United States

About the editor

Professor Mahmoud Elsabahy is the Vice Dean of the Badr University in Cairo (BUC) School of Biotechnology and the Head of BUC Science Academy (Cairo, Egypt). He is a professor of Pharmaceutical Technology and Nanomedicine. He has been the assistant director of a research facility at Texas A&M University (TX, USA, 2011–20). He was ranked in 2020 among top 1% scientists in the world in "Pharmacy and Pharmacology," as named by Stanford University World's top 2% scientists. He has completed MSc and PhD degrees from the Faculty of Pharmacy, University of Montreal "Pharmaceutical Nanotechnology" (Montreal, Canada). He contributed to 85 publications, all in international top profile peer-reviewed journals (e.g., *Nature Communications*, *Nano Letters*, and *Journal of the American Chemical Society*), book chapters, and US patents, and he is the principal investigator on several grant applications. Research interests include the rational design of pharmaceutical dosage forms and nanomedicine for various biomedical applications, for which he has received several national and international prestigious awards. In 2021, he won the "Gold Medal" in the International Exhibition of Inventions of Geneva. He was invited and sponsored by Luminex Co. (Austin, TX) and Bio-Rad Laboratories (Hercules, CA) as a keynote speaker at a 2017 meeting. During his talk, "Immunogenicity Profiling of Pharmaceutical Nanocarriers," at the xMAP Connect US Multiplexing Symposium (Cambridge, MA), he was among only nine experts from the United States.

Preface

Nanoscale objects, whether of biologic origin or synthetically created, are being developed for a variety of bionanotechnology diagnostic and pharmaceutical applications. The intent of this textbook is to provide the reader with a simplified overview on the assessment of the immunomodulatory effects of these materials, through detailed protocols and procedures for experimental measurements of biomarkers. At present, there are several valuable and well-written textbooks about nanoconstructs and immunotoxicity. However, there are no currently available books that guide researchers in academia and industry in the assessment of the immunotoxicity of nanoparticles and biomaterials, from concept to detailed protocols, for precise evaluation. Furthermore, no detailed description for processing and analyses of the intensively generated data from the multiplexing techniques are available.

The proposed book will provide a simplified overview on nanomaterials and the immune system, and on the assessment of the immunomodulatory effects of these materials, through detailed protocols and experimental measurements of biomarkers. The book will also cover the precautions that should be carefully considered during the assessment of particulate materials, and provide details on a newly developed algorithm, for data mining and analysis, as a simple and easy way to compare the immunotoxicity of various materials.

The subject of the book is of great interest to those who are working in industry and academia. It could be also utilized as course materials for postgraduate students in MSc and PhD levels in Chemistry, Pharmacy, Medicine, and Biomedical Science programs.

Acknowledgments

Life is a continuous learning journey and what makes this journey enjoyable are the people who share the gift of their time to support and mentor others. Thanks to everyone who strives to develop while helping others develop. Writing a book is much more tough than I expected. If this book was a success, this would not have been accomplished without the support of great mentors and colleagues that I have met throughout my career pathway.

To all the individuals I had the opportunity to learn from, to work with, or follow their success profile, I want to thank you for being the inspiration for the accomplishment of this work.

I owe an enormous debt of gratitude to Dr. Hassan El Kalla, Founder and Chairman of Badr University in Cairo, for his continuous support, guidance, and enormous inspiration.

I cannot thank enough Prof. Karen L. Wooley and Wooley Group at Texas A&M University (College Station, Texas, USA), for providing the knowledge, infrastructure, and sophisticated nanostructures that I could exploit to understand the effects of structures and compositions of nanomaterials on immunotoxicity, and to be able to write this book.

I am immensely grateful to Prof. Mostafa Kamal, President of Badr University in Cairo, for believing in me, for providing advice and assistance that has been immeasurably helpful both personally and academically.

I gratefully acknowledge Prof. Gamal Esmat, the past Vice President of Cairo University, for his kind support and guidance.

I would like to extend my sincere thanks to Prof. Ashraf Haider Ghaleb, President of Misr University for Science and Technology, Giza, Egypt, for providing guidance, support and advice.

I acknowledge with appreciation Prof. Jean-Christophe Leroux (ETH Zürich), my MSc and PhD mentor, and the one who gave me the first opportunity in my life to travel and study abroad and to get engaged in the field of nanomedicine.

I gratefully acknowledge Prof. Amr Elatraby, Vice President for Postgraduate Studies and International Relations of Badr University in Cairo, for his kind support and guidance.

I extend my acknowledgment to Dr. Noura G. Eissa (Zagazig University, Egypt), my colleague, who helped and encouraged me throughout the whole writing and editorial process of this book.

Nourhan K. Mohamed (Assiut University, Egypt) is also greatly acknowledged for assistance in editing this book.

I greatly acknowledge Elsevier, and Rafael G. Trombaco, Editorial Project Manager, for accepting my book proposal, and for providing all the necessary tools and personnel to successfully complete my mission, and for his wonderful editorial support and guidance.

Introduction

Nanomaterials and biomaterials have been implicated in a variety of biomedical applications, and their versatility and tunability allowed their emergence into several clinically viable commercial products. Toxicity and safety are routinely evaluated in vitro and in vivo via measurements of cellular cytotoxicity and lethality, respectively, in addition to other medical tests. Immunomodulation remains a critical threat that has raised special attention due to the severe consequences on healthy subjects if these effects are not assessed appropriately. Unintentional interactions between biomaterials and the immune system, although being life-threatening, may not be apparently observed by traditional toxicological assays. Biomarkers are exploited to evaluate the immunotoxicity of nanomaterials, particulates, and medical devices, and recent multiplexing techniques allowed measurements of up to 500 biomarkers in a few microliters of biological samples. However, measurements, data analysis, and interpretation should be carefully considered in this transdisciplinary area, as there are fundamental differences in physicochemical characteristics and biological behavior between particulate materials and low-molecular-weight molecules and drugs. Direct comparisons between the intensively generated data are nearly impossible. Adsorption and/or sequestration of biomarkers into biomaterials is also a challenge toward accurate assessment and appropriate data interpretation. This book provides a simplified overview on the potential interactions between biomaterials and particulates (nano- and micro-particles) and the immune system, and on the assessment of the immunomodulatory effects of these materials. In addition, detailed protocols and procedures for experimental measurements of biomarkers will be provided, together with precautions that should be carefully considered for handling and assessment of particulate materials. Furthermore, the application of the multiple analyte profiling index, a newly developed algorithm, for data mining and analysis will be demonstrated, as a simple and easy way to compare the intensively generated data and immunotoxicity of various materials.

Five key features are mainly covered in this book:

1. Potential interactions between nanomaterials and the immune system, and how structures and compositions of nanoconstructs influence the immune system.

2. Evaluation of the immunomodulatory effects of nanoparticles via multiplexing techniques.
3. Precautions during evaluation of immunotoxicity of particulate materials.
4. Data analysis and interpretation after measurements of the biomarkers.
5. Description of a newly developed algorithm for biomarkers data mining and analysis.

CHAPTER 1

Nanomaterials: classification, composition, and recent advances in synthesis

Ahmed S. Abo Dena[1,2], Omar A. Abdelaziz[1] and Ibrahim M. El-Sherbiny[1]
[1]Nanomedicine Laboratory, Center for Materials Science, Zewail City of Science and Technology, Giza, Egypt
[2]Pharmaceutical Chemistry Department, National Organization for Drug Control and Research (NODCAR), Giza, Egypt

1.1 Introduction to nanotechnology

Nanoscience is the study of materials in the nanoscale. Nano is a Greek word meaning tiny or very small. Nanotechnology is the field concerned with preparing and manipulating materials in that tiny scale. A nanometer is one-billionth of the meter. It is the smallest possible particle size compared to the atomic size that is measured in angstrom (i.e., one-tenth of the nanometer) (Saleh, 2020). Nanotechnology paved the doors for various applications because materials show completely different physical and chemical properties when prepared in nanosize. These alterations in the materials' properties were attributed to the changes happening in the electron energetics and confinement, opening the door to a whole new undiscovered world inside our real known world (Mazari et al., 2021).

Richard Adolf Zsigmondy coined the term "nanometer" in 1914. In 1959 the famous theoretical physicist, Professor Richard Feynman, introduced the promises of the nanotechnology field in a seminar titled "*There's Plenty of Room at the Bottom: An Invitation to Enter a New Field of Physics*." He explained the possibility of controlling and manipulating the material on its tiny scale for the sake of obtaining different desired physical and chemical material properties.

In 1974 Professor Norio Taniguchi from Tokyo Science University was the first to introduce the concept of nanotechnology and nanoscale science. Taniguchi's research work was directed to the preparation and processing of materials in the level of one single atom or molecule, which

Immunomodulatory Effects of Nanomaterials
DOI: https://doi.org/10.1016/B978-0-323-90604-3.00007-3

is well known today in the field of nanotechnology. Taniguchi's research group was the first to invent the atomic layer deposition (ALD) technique of thin-film preparation where the thickness of the film is just one single atom. As a matter of fact, the ALD technology is still used nowadays in microelectronics and silicon-based industries.

In the 1980s, a significant evolution in nanotechnology took place after the invention of the scanning tunneling microscope (STM). This type of microscope provided more control over the material preparation in addition to the manipulation ability in the scale of one single atom. For instance, an astonishing application was introduced by Eigler and Schweizer who were working at the famous American company IBM. They managed to manipulate Xenon atoms and push them to be adsorbed on a Nickel substrate to write the company logo by these single atoms (Fig. 1.1).

Nanomaterials have risen to prominence as an interesting new class of materials with a wide range of practical applications. The length of a

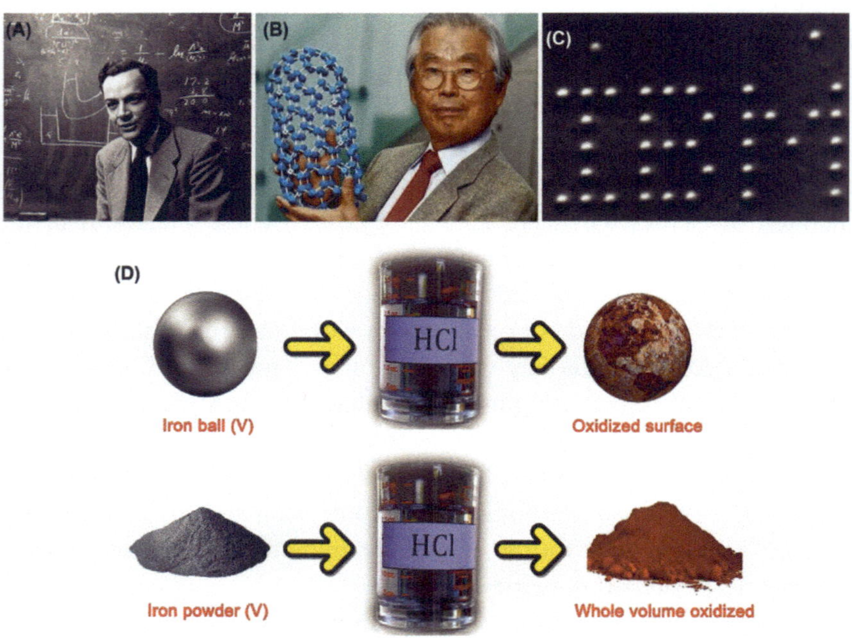

Figure 1.1 Nanomaterials. Professor Richard Feynman (A), Professor Norio Taniguchi (B), an STM image of the IBM logo written with single Xe atoms (C), and an illustration explaining the concept of increasing materials reactivity in the nanoscale due to the higher surface-area-to-volume ratio (D).

nanometer can be visualized by lining up 5 silicon atoms or 10 hydrogen atoms, which is equal to 1 nm. Materials are classified as nanomaterials if one or more of their dimensions are between 1 and 100 nm. It is difficult to pinpoint the exact timeline of human use of nanosized things. However, nanomaterials have a long history of use, and humans have inadvertently employed them for a variety of purposes for a long time. Asbestos nanofibers were used to strengthen ceramic mixes around 4500 years ago. PbS nanoparticles were known to the ancient Egyptians about 4000 years ago, and they were utilized in a hair coloring solution. Another intriguing example from the past is the Lycurgus Cup. It is a 4th century AD dichroic cup made by the Romans. In direct light, it has a jade-like appearance, yet in transmitted light, it has a ruby-like appearance. Color differences are visible based on the incident light (Kamaly et al., 2016). The presence of Ag and Au nanoparticles causes these color changes.

Nanomaterials are those appearing in the tiny scale below 100 nm. At that small size, these materials exhibit different quantum mechanical characteristics due to the changes in the energy of their electrons and also because of the electronic confinement in that limited size. One of the major properties of nanomaterials is the extensive high surface-area-to-volume ratio that results in a significant increase in the material reactivity. For instance, to understand the meaning of the surface area-to-volume ratio, two scenarios will be shown (Fig. 1.1). First, if we have a bulk metal ball of iron and if we put that ball in a solution of a strong corrosive acid for a while, then the surface of the ball will start to interact with the acid and oxidation occurs at the surface of the ball as shown in Fig. 1.1. We can actually return the ball to its first state if we just removed the oxidized surface that represents a small percentage of the overall ball volume. Second, if we smashed this bulky metal ball into billions of tiny pieces to obtain it as a powder and then added them to the same strong corrosive acid, then the observation here will be completely different. Almost all of the material particles will get oxidized in this case meaning that the material reactivity is directly dependent on the material unit size at the same volume.

Recently, nanomaterials contribute effectively to many different arms of industry and technology such as pharmaceutical sciences, medical sciences, electronics, cosmetics, food industry, agricultural applications, and almost every field related to material development. This wide range of applications grows up due to the favorable properties of nanomaterials such as their high reactivity, chemical and thermal stability, improved solubility, higher strength, and good mechanical properties. Therefore nanotechnology is a perfect example of innovative technology as it offers tailored nanoparticles with a huge potential for generating products with significantly better performance (Yan et al., 2017).

1.2 Terminology of nanotechnology

The precise meanings of nanomaterials and related terminologies are still up for debate. As a result, there is a lot of chances for the interpretation and classification of nanostructures. The term "nanomaterials" is difficult to define. Nanomaterials are described in a variety of manners in the literature owing to the unavailability of a clear description. Several scientists have used the term nanomaterial to describe anything with a dimension of a few nanometers or below a few tens of nanometers, while others used it to describe anything with a size of less than a micrometer. Nanomaterials' physical and chemical properties are determined by their particular composition, shape, and size. The impact of nanomaterials on human health and the environment is also influenced by their size, shape, and other characteristics. It is difficult to establish a single universal definition of nanomaterials, and a precise meaning is currently being debated in the research community. Here, we will describe some common terms used in nanotechnology.

Nanomanufacturing is the process of producing things at the nanoscale (a scale covering 1–100 nm) using either bottom-up or top-down methods. If a material has at least one dimension in the nanoscale, it is called a nanomaterial. In addition, when all of the dimensions of an object or particle are in the nanometer level, it is termed a nanoparticle. Moreover, the ratio of the length of the major axis to the width of the minor axis of a particle/object is referred to as the aspect ratio. Therefore a nanosphere is a nanoparticle with an aspect ratio of 1, while nanorods are nanoparticles with unequal short and long axes and an aspect ratio >1. The width of a nanorod must be in the nanoscale. Moreover, nanofibers are nanoobjects with two dimensions in the nanoscale and a significantly larger third dimension. The aspect ratio of nanowires is significantly higher than that of nanofibers. It is worth to mention that hollow nanofibers may be referred to as nanotubes. When different components with multiple different phase domains and at least one of these phases have at least one dimension in the nanoscale, this blend of materials is called nanocomposite (Aziz, 2020).

1.3 Unique properties of nanomaterials

Materials have completely different properties in the nanoscale compared to the bulk. Dividing the materials into very small pieces (i.e., nanostructures) makes the size-dependent properties more prominent. For instance, gold in the bulk is yellow while in the nanoscale it appears red or purple. In addition, boron does not show metallic properties in the bulk; however, in the nanoscale (2D sheets of borophene), it acts as a perfect metal. This change in the electronic properties is attributed to the decrease in size to the nanoscale. Moreover, the mechanical properties of materials can be enhanced significantly in the nanoscale due to the associated reduction in crystallographic defects which increases crystal perfection. Quantum mechanics govern the electronic properties of materials in the size range 1–10 nm. In this size range, the particles are called quantum dots whose properties strongly depend on their size and shape. The exciton diameter of the photogenerated electron–hole pair lies in the range of 1–10 nm. Therefore the optical properties of light absorption and/or emission of quantum dots can be manipulated by changing their particle size. Here, we will give a short account on the unique properties of materials in the nanoscale.

The reactive surface area of a bulk material exhibits a substantial increase when the material size is reduced down to the nanoscale. This property was briefly discussed in the introduction. Accordingly, the material's reactivity, adsorption capacity, catalytic efficiency, etc. may be significantly improved by reducing the material size to the nanoscale. In addition, the magnetic properties are strongly affected by size reduction due to the exhibited alterations in the electronic and quantum mechanical properties of the material. For instance, nonmagnetic materials can gain magnetic properties and be converted into magnetic materials at the nanoscale level.

Quantum effects are more explicitly pronounced in the nanoscale. However, the size at which the strength of these effects is maximum relies strongly on the type/nature of the material itself. Not only the previously mentioned properties but also the thermal and electrical properties of the materials can be changed in the nanoscale. Nanomaterials demonstrate extraordinary electrical and thermal conductivity, and the most common example, in this case, is graphene. Graphene also shows excellent mechanical properties comparable to that of diamond as an obvious evidence for improving the mechanical properties of materials at the nanoscale.

Furthermore, nanomaterials, especially 2D sheets, help in the dispersion of catalytic nanoparticles resulting in a pronounced improvement in the catalytic activity of these nanoparticles. On the biological/medical side, some materials exhibit strong biological activity (e.g., antiviral, antifungal, and antibacterial properties) in the nanoscale compared to the bulk state.

All the previously mentioned properties make nanomaterials potential candidates for different applications in many areas of science. In the following sections, we will classify nanomaterials and summarize some of the methods used for their synthesis (Aziz, 2020).

1.4 Classification of nanomaterials

There are many different ways to classify nanomaterials. They can be classified according to the approach of their syntheses, such as the bottom-up approach (i.e., starting from the atomic scale till reaching the nanoscale) and the top-down approach (i.e., starting from bulk material till reaching the nanoscale). They can also be classified according to the source or the origin of the material (i.e., either synthetic or natural). Another way of classification is considering the application. For example, in the case of biological applications, there are biologically safe materials (i.e., biocompatible and biodegradable) that are nontoxic and biologically toxic materials. Finally, nanomaterials can be classified according to their composition. The nanosystem parts can be held together by just a physical interaction or they are bound together via stronger and more stable chemical bonding (Saleh, 2020).

1.4.1 Polymeric nanoparticles

Polymer-based nanoparticles are one of the most essential classes of nanomaterials due to the wide range of polymers that can be prepared to serve almost all the fields related to material development such as medical applications (e.g., drug delivery, tissue engineering, and biosensors), agricultural applications, water treatment, and even cosmetics and healthcare products. Polymers can be classified into natural or synthetic, long chain or hyperbranched, and rare or abundant. Accordingly, the nanomaterials derived from them can be classified in the same manner.

Nanosized polymers are considered efficient carrier systems for any selected ingredient due to the wide range of polarity they offer (hydrophilic, hydrophobic, or even amphiphilic), in addition to being effective materials themselves.

Dendrimers are hyperbranched polymeric nanomaterials. They are considered a very promising type of nanoformulations due to the extensive existence of chemical functional groups on their surfaces. Dendrimers also have a huge surface area of interaction making them highly reactive materials, in addition to being potential carriers for various kinds of active substances. Dendrimers can be constructed from different kinds of polymers (synthetic or natural biocompatible/biodegradable polymers) making them advantageous nanosystems that can serve in a wide range of applications (Kamaly et al., 2016).

1.4.2 Nanoemulsions

An emulsion system is a simulation for heterogeneous solution systems. It provides a solution for the delivery of poorly soluble materials in specific solvent systems where the material will be suspended in the form of colloids throughout the solution without precipitation or aggregation. Nanoemulsions have the advantages of nanosize systems making the emulsion system more stable due to the large number of charges existing on the surface that keep the particles in continuous random repulsive motion.

A typical nanoemulsion system consists of two immiscible phases, oil and water, held together and stabilized by a surfactant or an emulsifier. Nanoemulsions can be classified into two main categories, single emulsion and double emulsion systems, each of which has two subcategories. The single emulsion can be simply oil in water (O/W), where the hydrophilic phase is the most dominant contributor and the oil phase is dispersed in it. On the other hand, the opposite situation is the second subcategory, water in oil (W/O), where water droplets are dispersed in the dominant oil phase. From the same perspective, the double emulsion can be oil in water in oil (O/W/O) or water in oil in water (W/O/W), having the advantage of being an amphiphilic system (provides the solubility of both hydrophilic and hydrophobic ingredients) (Marzuki et al., 2019).

Liposomes are a special type of hydrophobic nanomaterials and can be considered a subcategory of nanoemulsion systems. They consist of a bilayer of lipids with an aqueous layer enclosed inside making them a suitable carrier for both water and lipid-soluble ingredients. The main use of nanoliposomes is in drug delivery and cosmetic applications. Inside biological systems, the liposomes can carry the drug through the bloodstream with considerable stability and very efficient cellular penetration ability especially in brain drug delivery, as liposomes showed improved kinetics in penetrating the lipophilic blood–brain barrier. In cosmetics and transdermal drug delivery, nanoliposomes are widely used due to their suitable tendency to the nature of the skin, in addition, being in the nanosize gives them more advantages, such as higher loading capacity for the selected ingredients, higher reactivity, and better kinetic profile.

Another subclass of nanoemulsion systems is niosomes that recently found a wide range of applications compared to liposomes. The main difference between liposomes and niosomes is that niosomes are formed of nonionic surfactants, while liposomes are composed of lipids. Niosomes may be unilamellar, bilamellar, or multilamellar depending on the number of layers of which they are formed. Similar to liposomes, the presence of more than one layer provides the advantage of amphiphilicity that allows for the delivery of both hydrophilic and hydrophobic drugs. The concept of nanoemulsification can be applied to prepare different kinds of nanomaterials including polymeric nanoparticles. This depends on the hydrophilicity of the used materials and the nature of the solvent (Singh et al., 2017).

1.4.3 Inorganic nanoparticles

Inorganic nanoparticles represent an essential branch of nanoformulations due to their interesting properties and their wide range of applications that allow their effective contribution to the development of material science. The inorganic category of nanoparticles includes, for example, but is not limited to, metallic nanoparticles, magnetic nanoparticles, carbon nanotubes, graphene oxide, and mesoporous silica (Lv et al., 2019).

As materials in the nanoscale show different physical and chemical properties, metals such as gold and silver show completely different optical activity when they are prepared in the form of metal nanoparticles. The unique optical behavior of silver and gold nanoparticles makes them potential optical sensors that detect certain existence of materials and reflect the change in the form of optical change [change in their light interaction (absorption and transmission of light)] that could be detected quantitatively.

For instance, silver nanoparticles are used as an optical sensor for the detection of ammonia in solutions, which is a highly important application for liver functions testing. Another important application of silver and gold nanoparticles is their antimicrobial activity. Due to their small size and high surface positive charge, they show great ability to get into various kinds of bacterial cells and kill them in a very efficient way, so they paved the way for a new era of nanomaterial-based antibacterial agents.

Another type of inorganic nanomaterial is magnetic nanoparticles. Materials can be classified according to their magnetic behavior into two major categories, namely, paramagnetic materials that respond to applied external magnetic fields and diamagnetic materials that do not have any response toward magnets. A new generation of paramagnetic materials, called superparamagnetic materials, has gripped the attention of researchers recently. The reason behind their modified magnetic properties is that the electronic orbitals of the prepared material are highly aligned in one direction making the net magnetic moment higher than that of the ordinary paramagnetic material. Magnetite (Fe_3O_4), an iron oxide, can be prepared in the nanosize and in a highly crystalline form for the sake of obtaining superparamagnetic properties. Nowadays, researchers actually have developed several methods for the preparation of superparamagnetic iron oxide nanoparticles (SPIONs) and utilized them in so many applications (Fig. 1.2).

In addition to the previously mentioned properties of nanomaterials including the high surface area of interaction and high reactivity, SPIONs are promising potential drug carriers due to their flexible surface chemistry and the expression of charges over their surface. They can be coated with various kinds of polymers and then be loaded with different kinds of ingredients. Besides the superparamagnetic property that make SPIONs highly responsive to magnets, they also exhibit metallic properties and good optical and thermal behaviors. As a result, SPIONs are used recently in biosensors and hyperthermia-based cancer therapy (Aziz, 2020).

1.4.4 Carbonaceous nanomaterials

These are a special class of nanomaterials consisting of one thin layer of carbon atoms combined together chemically. Examples of carbonaceous nanomaterials are graphene, fullerenes, and carbon nanotubes (CNTs) (Fig. 1.2). Graphene and CNTs show improved mechanical properties in terms of stress—strain behavior and strength factor (stronger than steel). In addition to the previously mentioned mechanical properties, carbonaceous nanomaterials demonstrate metallic properties (excellent electrical and thermal conductivity) making them potential materials for many applications such as automobile and airplanes manufacture, small electronic and digital devices, and also modified steel and building materials. It is worth to mention that CNTs can be imagined as a 2D carbon sheet rolled about itself. They can be either single-walled CNTs (SWCNTs) in the form of

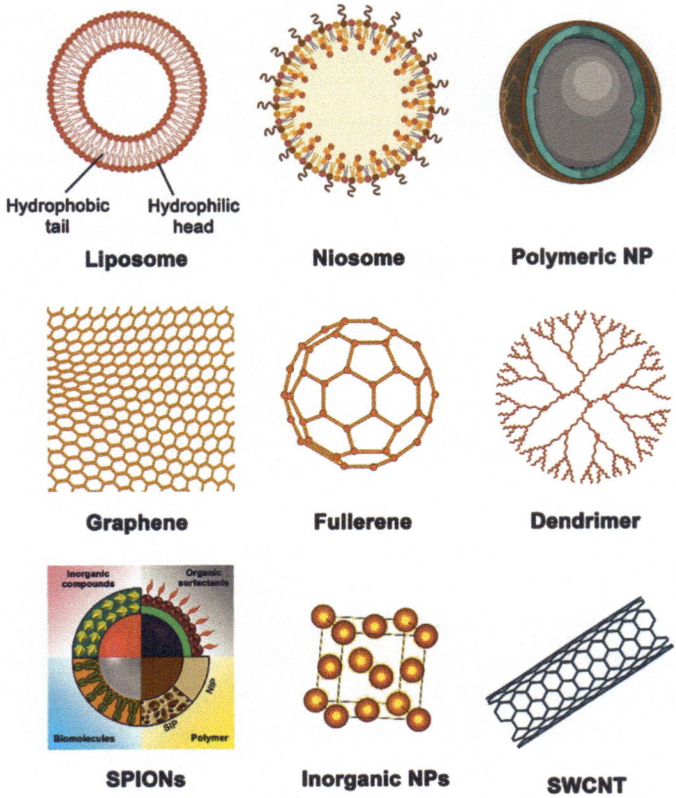

Figure 1.2 Examples for the different classes of nanomaterials. The possible manners of modifying the surface of SPIONs (the four basic SPIONs colors are depicted in the central nanoparticle; *SIP*, surface-imprinted polymer; *NIP*, nonimprinted polymer) are shown.

only one carbon cylinder or multiwalled CNTs (MWCNTs) in the form of two or more concentric cylinders (Shah & Tali, 2016).

Among the carbonaceous nanomaterials are 3D structures called fullerenes or buckyballs. These structures usually consist of hollow cages of sixty or more atoms. Fullerenes are considered excellent materials for drug delivery applications, and they can be easily prepared by arc discharge between two carbon electrodes in an inert atmosphere.

1.5 Nanomaterial synthesis

Recently, various methods of synthesis of nanomaterials have been developed. These methods can be classified in different ways such as chemical and physical methods, high-energy and low-energy methods, and small-scale production and large-scale production methods. Yet, researchers follow two main approaches to synthesize nanomaterials, namely, the top-down and the bottom-up approaches (Fig. 1.3). In Table 1.1, different kinds and synthesis techniques are presented with a comparison between their advantages and disadvantages (Mazari et al., 2021).

1.6 Characterization of nanomaterials

1.6.1 Stability and surface chemistry

Zeta potential is a technique that measures the stability of the prepared nanomaterials by measuring the particles' surface charge. Nanoparticles usually have a higher charge on the surface compared to the bulk particles due to the higher surface-area-to-volume ratio for the same material (i.e., the expression of the charge on the surface is higher). As a result, the prepared particles show high stability in solution forms. This high charge at the surface keeps the particles in continuous electrostatic repulsion with one another and enhances the long-term stability of the prepared nanoparticles suspension. Table 1.2 shows the relation between the ζ potential value and nanoparticles system stability (Fofaria et al., 2016).

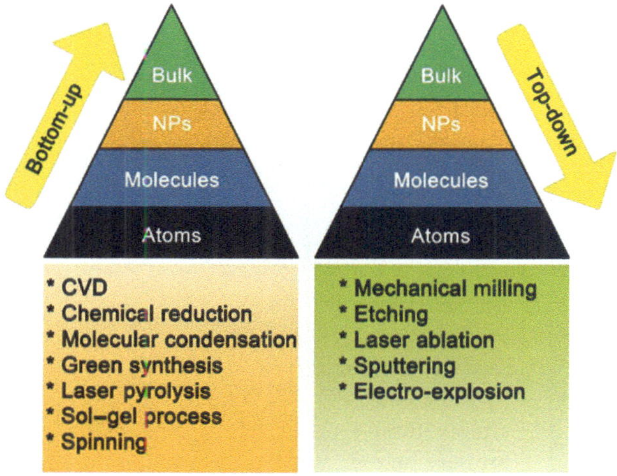

Figure 1.3 Synthesis of nanomaterials. The two main approaches used to synthesize nanomaterials and examples of their subapproaches.

Table 1.1 Common methods used for synthesizing nanomaterials and some of their advantages and drawbacks.

Method	Description	Advantages	Disadvantages
Mechanical milling	A top-down approach to produce a fine powder from a starting bulk material It requires a high-energy source (usually a traditional mechanical source) of milling in addition to a milling medium	• Production of fine nanopowder down to 20 nm • Suitability for large-scale production and long-time operation • Relatively affordable effectiveness	• Production of a wide range of sizes in the same batch • High noise and distributing vibrations
Coprecipitation	A chemical bottom-up approach mainly used for the synthesis of metal and magnetic nanoparticles. Firstly, the salt precursor of the metal gets dissolved in an aqueous solution to obtain the metal ions; secondly, the metal ions are reduced and precipitated to form nanoparticles. Precipitation may be induced by pH changes, temperature/pressure raising, and the existence of a suitable reducing agent	• The produced size can be controlled by varying parameters such as temperature, pH, salt concentration, and capping agents • Low-energy and cost-effective technique Fast technique	• Efficient only for small-scale production • Gives a wide range of sizes, the resultant batch is not highly uniform • Further purification is needed because other ingredients are precipitated in addition to the metal nanoparticles

(Continued)

Table 1.1 (Continued)

Method	Description	Advantages	Disadvantages
Physical and chemical vapor deposition (PVD and CVD)	A bottom-up technique for the formation of thin films. They are also used in further coating for the already prepared nanomaterials or during preparation (in situ preparation) Briefly, the deposited material is vaporized and then moved to rotating vacuum champers allowing the deposition/ condensation to occur in the form of thin (nano) film	• PVD is a green method with no possible toxicity • Very efficient technique for the outer polymeric coating for the nanomaterial	• CVP might be toxic • Not scalable
Hydrothermal method	A bottom-up physical approach mainly used to form crystalline nanomaterials such as metals and magnetic nanoparticles. The induction of crystallization needs extremely high temperature and pressure to obtain highly crystalline and pure nanoparticles	• Produces highly homogenous and uniform nanoparticles • Produces highly pure crystalline materials as most of the impurities cannot withstand the used high temperature and pressure	• Safety issues due to the extremely high temperature and pressure • Not cost effective (needs specific autoclaves that withstands the harsh conditions)

(Continued)

Table 1.1 (Continued)

Method	Description	Advantages	Disadvantages
		• Factors such as size, degree of crystallinity, and morphology can be optimized	
Sol–gel	A wet chemical bottom-up approach to produce solid nanoparticles in the form of colloids dispersed homogenously in a solution phase. It consists of two main parts, sol (solution phase) and the gel, which is the integrated network of nanoparticles	• A low-energy, cost- and time-effective method • Produces nanoparticles with different size ranges	• The used organic solvents are toxic • Not suitable for large-scale production
Inert gas condensation	A physical bottom-up approach to produce powdered nanoparticles. The particles precursor is firstly dissolved in a certain solvent, and then the solvent starts to evaporate carrying the dissolved particles. In the presence of inert cool gas in the surroundings, the particles start to condensate in the nanosize at the cold surface	• Green method • Can produce large amounts of particles based on the capacity of the used device (condenser)	• Time consuming • Not cost effective

(Continued)

Table 1.1 (Continued)

Method	Description	Advantages	Disadvantages
Laser ablation	A top-down physical approach that uses laser ablation technique. Nanoparticles in the form of colloids are prepared via induction by an external laser beam. The energy of the laser beam stimulates the nucleation growth of the nanoparticles when the beam hits the solid precursor in a solvent or gas system	• Green method (no need for chemicals or reducing agents) • No toxicity occurs, so it is highly recommended for the medical application, cosmetics, and food industry • Produce highly pure and homogenous nanoparticles	• Expensive Not efficient for large-scale production due to its low yield • The laser source requires continuous maintenance

1.6.2 Particle size measurement and polydispersity

It is highly essential and critical to measure the particle size of the prepared nanoparticles (i.e., average particle diameter) as it gives an indication of the system stability, dispersity, homogeneity, and also reactivity. The smaller the prepared particles, the higher is their reactivity. Dynamic light scattering technique is one of the spectroscopic techniques that gives a description of the particle size and the distribution of the sizes in a nanoparticle sample suspension. In a word, the closer the particle size to the nanoscale (10–200 nm), the more stable they are, with higher reactivity, and less aggregation possibility. It is highly needed for the prepared particles to have the previously mentioned properties of stability and reactivity, as they are preferred from the industrial point of view as they add more value to the resultant products from the material development perspective (Alshamsan et al., 2018).

Table 1.2 Relation between the values of the particle surface charge and the stability of the nanoparticle system.

Zeta potential range (mV)		Stability of the nanoparticles system
From	**To**	
+5	−5	Unstable with fast aggregation rate
+20	−20	Short-term stability with slow aggregation rate
+30	−30	Stable system
+60	−60	Perfectly stable system

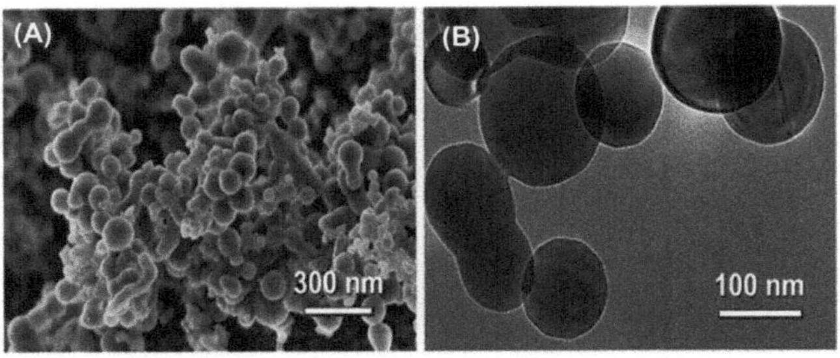

Figure 1.4 Example for 3D SEM image (A) and 2D TEM image (B) of nanoparticles. *Reproduced from Shao, D., Smolianova, I., Tang, D., & Zhang, L. (2017). Novel core–shell structured Si/S-doped-carbon composite with buffering voids as high performance anode for Li-ion batteries.* RSC Advances *7(5), 2407–2414. https://doi.org/10.1039/C6RA26247C, with permission from the Royal Society of Chemistry.*

1.6.3 Electron microscopy and imaging

This type of microscopy gives an accurate indication of the particle size, shape, and morphology. Also, it gives an overview of the sample homogeneity (i.e., how close the size of the particles is with respect to one another). There are actually several types of electron microscopy that differ in the mechanism of operation and give different images from different perspectives (Fig. 1.4) (Shao et al., 2017).

The first type of electron microscopes is the scanning electron microscope (SEM). In this technique, an electron energy range from 1 to 30 kV is directed toward the sample, and then the reflected and scattered beams of electrons are used to draw a three-dimensional image showing the morphology and topology of the particles' surfaces clearly. Second, transmission electron microscopy (TEM) is considered a relatively high-energy technique compared to the previously mentioned SEM technique. In TEM, a high-energy electron (60–600 kV) is used for imaging, meaning that the wavelength of the beam is short enough to penetrate the prepared nanoparticles and then get reflected after penetration creating a two-dimensional image for the particle and showing what is existing inside the particle as well (Ealia & Saravanakumar, 2017).

1.6.4 Ultraviolet—visible spectroscopy

This kind of spectroscopic technique can be used to characterize both metallic and organic nanomaterials qualitatively and quantitatively. Each metal has a specific absorption through the light spectrum. Ultraviolet—visible (UV—VIS) spectroscopy is an efficient way for the determination of metal formation and the metal purity as well. Some metal nanoparticles such as silver and gold can be used as optical sensors by applying UV—VIS spectroscopy for detection.

1.7 Concluding remarks and future avenue

Nanomaterials and technologies is an interdisciplinary, one-of-a-kind branch of study that has a substantial impact on society's long-term sustainability. It is a rapidly developing field with numerous unique applications in electronics, energy, medicine, information technology, and other fields. Nanomaterials have endless potential for tuning electrical, optical, chemical, mechanical, and magnetic properties, allowing them to revolutionize a wide range of commercial nanotechnologies. They have a significant promise for improving health by boosting the safety and efficiency of nanomedicines/nanodevices to treat any condition. The ability of nanodevices to assess the characteristics and performance of nanomaterials at the nanoscale reliably and reproducibly is critical for progress in this sector. Highly advanced tools with nanoscale precision metrology are necessary to ensure the accuracy of nanosystem measurements. As a result, nanometrological tools and techniques, as well as advances in nanomaterials and technology, are critical. Nanoindentation, ellipsometry, scanning probe microscopies, and other state-of-the-art instrumentation are all helping to a better understanding of many aspects of nanomaterials and technology. However, for more sophisticated future applications, nanoscale accuracy and investigation must be increased. As a result, nanometrological tools and procedures are being integrated into new nanotechnology-based materials and devices. These are the most important aspects of nanotechnology's success (Punia et al., 2021).

To support effective nanomanufacturing for commercialization, new and innovative processes, tools, and infrastructure will be required. Existing nanometrological tools are approaching their resolution and accuracy limits and hence are unlikely to match future nanotechnology or nanomanufacturing requirements. Some unique, cutting-edge techniques are required, such as tip-enhanced Raman spectroscopy, which can produce substantially better resolution values and gives a nine-order-of-magnitude improvement in Raman signal and lateral resolution. Nanolevel science and technology will demand similar types of new and more advanced approaches in the near future. Still, more innovative novel ideas are needed to improve nanometrology measurement systems. Simultaneously, for certifying, calibrating, and checking nanometrology instruments, it is critical to construct standard samples and standardized procedures for measurements in the nanometer scale, which enable the transfer of the units' properties and response from the nanometer to the macroscopic scale without any appreciable loss of accuracy. Revolutionary techniques to nanometrology and apparatus for property measurement are critical for civilizations' long-term survival.

References

Alshamsan, A., Kazi, M., Badran, M. M., & Alanazi, F. K. (2018). Role of alternative lipid excipients in the design of self-nanoemulsifying formulations for fenofibrate: Characterization, in vitro dispersion, digestion and ex vivo gut permeation studies. *Frontiers in Pharmacology*, 9. Available from https://doi.org/10.3389/fphar.2018.01219.

Aziz, O. A. A. (2020). Superparamagnetic iron oxide nanoparticles (SPIONs): Preparation and recent applications. *Journal of Nanotechnology Advanced Material, 8*, 21–29.

Ealia, S. A. M., & Saravanakumar, M. (2017). A review on the classification, characterisation, synthesis of nanoparticles and their application. In *IOP conference series: Materials science and engineering*.

Fofaria, N. M., Qhattal, H. S. S., Liu, X., & Srivastava, S. K. (2016). Nanoemulsion formulations for anti-cancer agent piplartine—Characterization, toxicological, pharmacokinetics and efficacy studies. *International Journal of Pharmaceutics, 498*(1–2), 12–22. Available from https://doi.org/10.1016/j.ijpharm.2015.11.045.

Kamaly, N., Yameen, B., Wu, J., & Farokhzad, O. C. (2016). Degradable controlled-release polymers and polymeric nanoparticles: Mechanisms of controlling drug release. *Chemical Reviews, 116*(4), 2602–2663. Available from https://doi.org/10.1021/acs.chemrev.5b00346.

Lv, J., Christie, P., & Zhang, S. (2019). Uptake, translocation, and transformation of metal-based nanoparticles in plants: Recent advances and methodological challenges. *Environmental Science Nano, 6*(1), 41–59. Available from https://doi.org/10.1039/C8EN00645H.

Marzuki, N. H. C., Wahab, R. A., & Hamid, M. A. (2019). An overview of nanoemulsion: Concepts of development and cosmeceutical applications. *Biotechnology and Biotechnological Equipment, 33*(1), 779–797. Available from https://doi.org/10.1080/13102818.2019.1620124.

Mazari, S. A., Ali, E., Abro, R., Khan, F. S. A., Ahmed, I., Ahmed, M., Nizamuddin, S., Siddiqui, T. H., Hossain, N., Mubarak, N. M., & Shah, A. (2021). Nanomaterials: Applications, waste-handling, environmental toxicities, and future challenges—A review. *Journal of Environmental Chemical Engineering, 9*(2), 105028. Available from https://doi.org/10.1016/j.jece.2021.105028.

Punia, P., Bharti, M. K., Chalia, S., Dhar, R., Ravelo, B., Thakur, P., & Thakur, A. (2021). Recent advances in synthesis, characterization, and applications of nanoparticles for contaminated water treatment—A review. *Ceramics International*, *47*(2), 1526–1550. Available from https://doi.org/10.1016/j.ceramint.2020.09.050.

Saleh, T. A. (2020). Nanomaterials: Classification, properties, and environmental toxicities. *Environmental Technology and Innovation*, 20. Available from https://doi.org/10.1016/j.eti.2020.101067.

Shah, K. A., & Tali, B. A. (2016). Synthesis of carbon nanotubes by catalytic chemical vapour deposition: A review on carbon sources, catalysts and substrates. *Materials Science in Semiconductor Processing*, *41*, 67–82. Available from https://doi.org/10.1016/j.mssp.2015.08.013.

Shao, D., Smolianova, I., Tang, D., & Zhang, L. (2017). Novel core–shell structured Si/S-doped-carbon composite with buffering voids as high performance anode for Li-ion batteries. *RSC Advances*, 7(5), 2407–2414. Available from https://doi.org/10.1039/C6RA26247C.

Singh, Y., Meher, J. G., Raval, K., Khan, F. A., Chaurasia, M., Jain, N. K., & Chourasia, M. K. (2017). Nanoemulsion: Concepts, development and applications in drug delivery. *Journal of Controlled Release*, *252*, 28–49. Available from https://doi.org/10.1016/j.jconrel.2017.03.008.

Yan, X., Tong, Z., Chen, Y., Mo, Y., Feng, H., Li, P., Qu, X., & Jin, S. (2017). Bioresponsive materials for drug delivery based on carboxymethyl chitosan/poly (γ-glutamic acid) composite microparticles. *Marine Drugs*, *15*(5). Available from https://doi.org/10.3390/md15050127.

CHAPTER 2

Applications of nanoengineered therapeutics and vaccines: special emphasis on COVID-19*

Nourhan Mohamed[1], Mostafa A. Hamad[2], Ashraf H. Ghaleb[3,4], Gamal Esmat[5,6] and Mahmoud Elsabahy[3,7]
[1]Department of Microbiology and Immunology, Faculty of Pharmacy, Sphinx University, Assiut, Egypt
[2]Department of Surgery, Faculty of Medicine, Assiut University, Assiut, Egypt
[3]Misr University for Science and Technology, 6th of October City, Giza, Egypt
[4]Department of Surgery, Faculty of Medicine, Cairo University, Cairo, Egypt
[5]Badr University in Cairo, Badr City, Cairo, Egypt
[6]Department of Hepatogastroenterology and Infectious Diseases, Faculty of Medicine, Cairo University, Cairo, Egypt
[7]School of Biotechnology and Science Academy, Badr University in Cairo, Badr City, Cairo, Egypt

2.1 Coronavirus disease-2019

Coronavirus disease-2019 (COVID-19) is a rapidly spreading disease in all of the six continents since it first appeared in Wuhan, China, in December 2019, leading to a pandemic, reporting 1,38,76,441 confirmed cases and 5,93,087 confirmed deaths to date, according to the World Health Organization (WHO) (Coronavirus Disease COVID-19 Pandemic, 2021). It is caused by the newly evolved strain of coronavirus, severe acute respiratory syndrome coronavirus-2 (SARS-CoV-2), according to the international virus classification commission (Coronaviridae Study Group of the International Committee on Taxonomy of Viruses, 2020). SARS-CoV-2 is highly contagious, probably due to spreading via asymptomatic-infected individuals and the long incubation periods of up to 24 days (Chan et al., 2020; Rothe et al., 2020). Previous severe outbreaks induced by other members of the same corona family were associated with SARS in China in 2003, which was caused by the severe acute respiratory syndrome coronavirus (SARS-CoV), and middle east

* Information regarding diagnosis and therapeutic protocols for the management of COVID-19 are continuously changing. Details included in this chapter are updated based on the information available at the time of writing the chapter, but may not present the current situation.

Immunomodulatory Effects of Nanomaterials
DOI: https://doi.org/10.1016/B978-0-323-90604-3.00003-6

respiratory syndrome (MERS) infection in Saudi Arabia in 2012, which was triggered by the MERS-coronavirus (CoV) (Coronaviridae Study Group of the International Committee on Taxonomy of Viruses, 2020).

2.2 Morphological structure and genome

SARS-CoV-2 belongs to the Coronaviridae family that comprises enveloped viruses encapsulating positive-sense, single-stranded RNA. The genome of the SARS-CoV-2 is c. 30 kb in size (Fig. 2.1) (Chan et al., 2020; Aust, 2019). Nonstructural proteins 1–16 are encoded by open

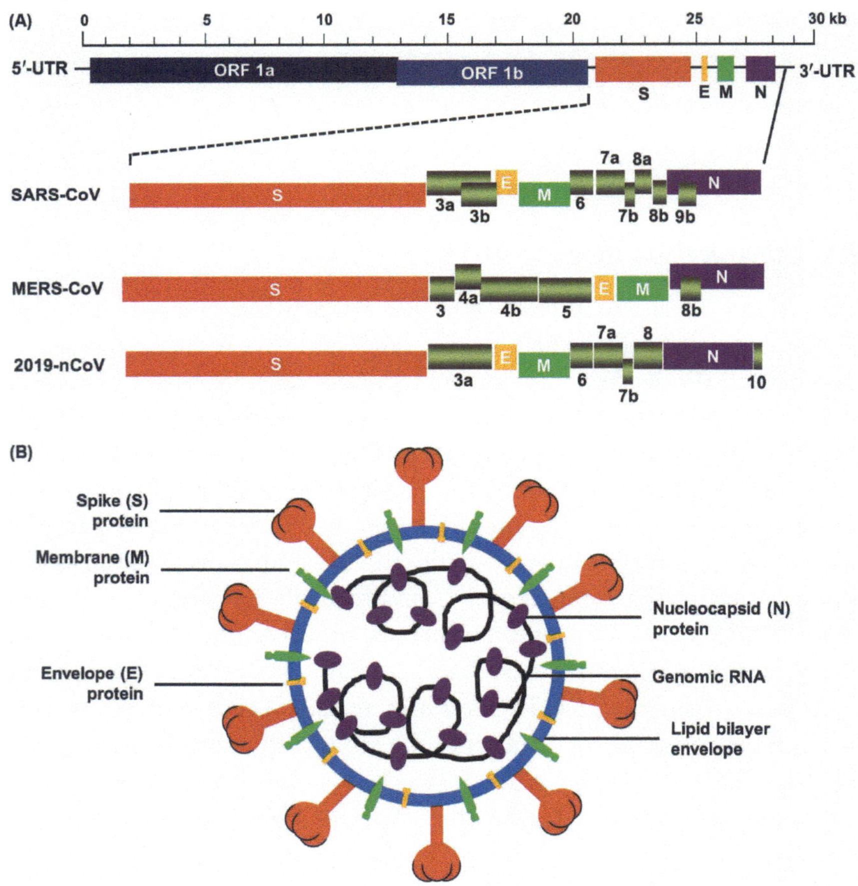

Figure 2.1 SARS-CoV-2 virus. Schematic diagram of genomic organization (A) and virion structure (B) of SARS-CoV, MERS-CoV, and SARS-CoV-2, and their major structural proteins. *From Wang, N., Shang, J., Jiang, S., & Du, L. (2020). Subunit vaccines against emerging pathogenic human coronaviruses.* Frontiers in Microbiology, 28, *298.*

reading frame (ORF) 1a/b at the 5′-end, followed by structural proteins (surface spike (S) glycoprotein, envelope (E), membrane (M), and nucleocapsid (N)), which are encoded by other ORFs at the 3′-end (Huang et al., 2020). Spike proteins S are club-shaped projections that play a key role in viral cell entry, as they bind to the angiotensin-converting enzymes (ACE2) receptors on the host cell surfaces through a subunit called receptor binding domain, followed by activation by transmembrane serine protease 2 (TMPRSS2), a transmembrane protease protein (Hoffmann et al., 2020). The receptor-binding domain is a highly antigenic part of the S protein of SARS-CoV-2, that is responsible for binding with ACE2 receptors on the host cells (Tai et al., 2020). The M and E proteins are necessary for virus assembly (de Haan & Rottier, 2005; Surya et al., 2015). The N protein is one of the major structural proteins of the virus that is involved in the transcription and replication of the viral RNA and interference with the cell cycle processes of the host cells (Huang et al., 2020).

2.3 Clinical presentation, radiological features, and laboratory investigations

COVID-19 may be presented clinically as mild, moderate, or severe. Symptoms presented include fever, fatigue, dry cough, anorexia, myalgia, dyspnea, and, in some of the cases, diarrhea, nausea, and vomiting (Huang et al., 2020; Wang, Cao, et al., 2020; Wang, Hu, et al., 2020; Wang, Wang, et al., 2020). In one study, it was found that c. 81% of people testing positive for SARS-CoV-2 are asymptomatic or have mild symptoms (Ing et al., 2020). Clinical diagnosis of COVID-19 is mainly based on epidemiological history, clinical manifestations, and several investigations, such as real-time quantitative polymerase chain reaction, computed tomography (CT) scan, and immune identification technologies. Chest CT shows bilateral multilobar consolidation "ground glass appearance" in the lung (Chung et al., 2020; Wang, Cao, et al., 2020; Wang, Hu, et al., 2020; Wang, Wang, et al., 2020). Laboratory investigations performed on COVID-19 patients demonstrated decreased albumin, high C-reactive protein, lymphopenia, high erythrocyte sedimentation rate, prolonged prothrombin time, and elevated lactate dehydrogenase, in most of the patients (Rodriguez-Morales et al., 2020; Wang, Cao, et al., 2020; Wang, Hu, et al., 2020; Wang, Wang, et al., 2020). High levels of proinflammatory cytokines and chemokines including IL-1β, IL-2, IL-6, IL-7, interferon-γ, G-CSF, IP-10, MCP-1, MIP-1a, TNF-α, CXCL10, and CCL2, were all observed in the COVID-19 severe cases, which is called "cytokine storm," that is one of the mechanisms of the acute respiratory distress syndrome. Cytokine storm can initiate viral sepsis and lung injury, thus leading to other complications, including, respiratory failure, shock, organ failure, and potentially death (Bani-Sadr et al., 2020; Huang et al., 2020; Kuppalli & Rasmussen, 2020; Ruscitti et al., 2020; Sun et al., 2020; Xu et al., 2020; Zhang et al., 2020). This massive rise in cytokines and chemokines levels indicates an increased activity of T helper 1 cells (Th1). A rise in antiinflammatory cytokines, such as IL-4 and IL-10, were also observed in COVID-19 infection, which are T helper 2 cells (Th2) cytokines, indicating an increased activity of these cells (Zhang et al., 2020). Higher risk of infection was observed in older age, male gender, and in individuals with comorbid conditions, such as hypertension, cardiovascular diseases, diabetes, malignancy, and, less commonly, cerebrovascular diseases, chronic obstructive pulmonary disease, chronic kidney disease, chronic liver disease, and human immunodeficiency virus infections (Chung et al., 2020; Wang, Cao, et al., 2020; Wang, Hu, et al., 2020; Wang, Wang, et al., 2020). These risk groups account for the majority of severe diseases and fatalities to date. Nucleic acid amplification tests using real-time polymerase chain reactions are considered as the most common effective method for detecting the virus, with a sensitivity of 50%–79%, depending on the protocol used, sample type, and the number of clinical specimens collected (Corman et al., 2020). The viral genes targeted so far include N, E, S, and RNA-dependent RNA polymerase (RdRP) genes (World Health Organization, Laboratory Testing for Coronavirus Disease 2019 (COVID-19) in Suspected Human Cases: Interim Guidance, 2020). The RdRP protein is essentially encoded in the genome of RNA viruses to catalyze the synthesis of the RNA complementary strand. Viral serological testing is an effective means of diagnosis of SARS-CoV-2 infection. The positive rate and titer variance of the human immunoglobulin IgG are higher than those of IgM in COVID-19 patients. The IgM-positive rate increases slightly at first and then decreases over time; whereas, the IgG-positive rate increases and remains higher than IgM (Zhou et al., 2020). Previous knowledge from literature indicated that neutralizing antibodies secreted by the host's body against SARS-CoV-2 are protective, but they last for a limited time (Hoffmann et al., 2020). However, for the vaccine to be effective, it should induce long-lasting immunity. T memory cells (i.e., $CD4^+$ and $CD8^+$ cells) are needed to pose this long-lasting effect, and previous studies that investigated specimens from COVID-19 patients found $CD4^+$ and $CD8^+$ cells that fight against infection (Grifoni et al., 2020; Hoffmann et al., 2020). Globally, there is a trend to screen people for their immunocompetence toward COVID-19, to allow healthcare workers who have antibodies in their blood to return to work in high-risk situations. Identifying individuals with antibodies in their blood can be beneficial for use of their convalescent plasma for the treatment of people with severe COVID-19 infections, to boost their ability to fight the virus. However, experts worry that widespread antibody screening may give those who test positive a false sense of security.

2.4 Therapeutic attempts

The development of effective medical therapeutic strategies against the SARS-CoV-2 virus is a critical initiative to control the spread of COVID-19 and to reduce the burden on the economy and health services. Therapeutic strategies include symptomatic support (e.g., antipyretics) and administration of steroids, antiviral drugs, immunomodulators, vaccines, and convalescent plasma. Corticosteroids are commonly used to manage acute respiratory distress syndromes due to their antiinflammatory effects. However, their immune-suppressive effects have discouraged their use in patients with viral infections, and their use in COVID-19 is controversial (Bani-Sadr et al., 2020; Fadel et al., 2020; Lu et al., 2020). RECOVERY trial, a randomized trial investigating whether treatment with either lopinavir-ritonavir, hydroxychloroquine, corticosteroids, azithromycin, convalescent plasma, or tocilizumab prevents death in patients with COVID-19, was conducted on total 12,000 subjects. In this trial, 2104 patients were assigned to the dexamethasone group and 4321 patients were assigned to the standard care group (ClinicalTrials.gov: NCT04381936). Results indicated that dexamethasone could be beneficial for severely ill COVID-19 patients who required either mechanical ventilation or supplemental oxygen support. Dexamethasone reduced mortality and decreased time of hospitalization among these patients when compared to the standard care group. However, no benefits were observed for mildly and moderately infected patients who are not requiring oxygen support Covid-19 Treatment Guidelines (2021). In this section, we will briefly introduce some of the commonly utilized strategies for the potential treatment of COVID-19 and immunization against the virus (Fig. 2.2). Then, in the following sections, we will provide an

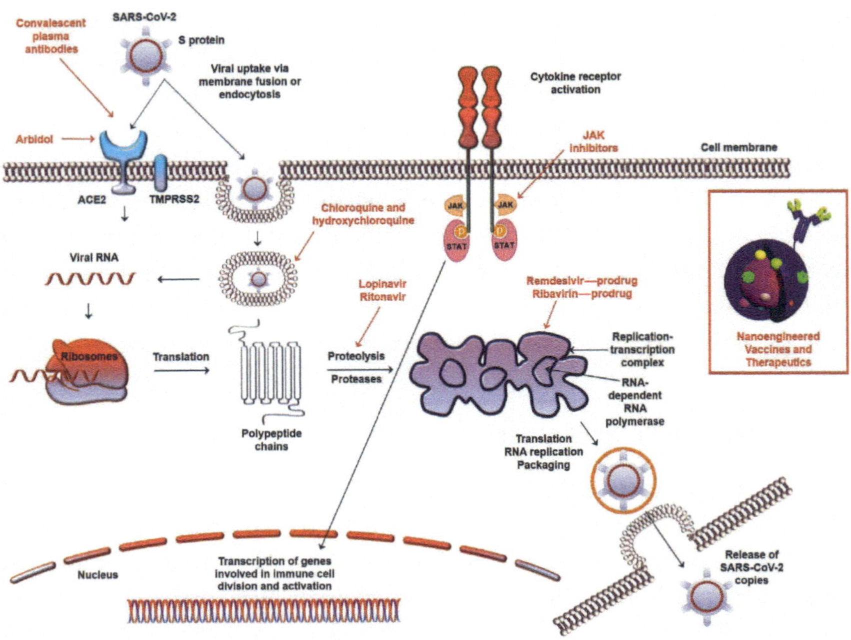

Figure 2.2 Demonstration of the antiviral drugs that are exploited in the management of COVID-19 and their underlying mechanisms of action. SARS-CoV-2 binds to ACE2 receptors on the host cell surface, with the aid of TMPRSS2 transmembrane protein, or the virus may fuse with the cell membrane and release the viral RNA into the cytoplasm. SARS-CoV-2 utilizes ribosomes to synthesize polypeptides that are being cleaved later by proteases into nonstructural proteins. In addition, the virus replicates its own RNA using the host cell machinery and utilizes RNA-dependent RNA polymerase to synthesize a copy of its RNA, besides several other cellular organelles and enzymes to continue translating the other structural proteins and transcribing the + RNA strands. Chloroquine and hydroxychloroquine mechanisms of action are not clearly known, although it is assumed that they inhibit viral entry, transport, postentry events and possibly increase the pH of endosomes and lysosomes. Remdesivir is a prodrug of GS-441524, and it resembles viral nucleoside. After viral entry, viral RNA initiates replication with the aid of RNA-dependent RNA polymerase. GS-441524 is incorporated into viral RNA rendering it defective. Ribavirin is a prodrug, which after being metabolized, it mimics RNA nucleotides, thus ultimately producing defective viral RNA. Lopinavir and ritonavir are protease inhibitors that prevent the formation of viral structural proteins. Arbidol inhibits membrane fusion of the virus with the host cells. JAK inhibitors block cytokine-mediated signals via the JAK-STAT pathway. Upon binding of cytokines to their receptors, JAK proteins initiate phosphorylation of STAT proteins rendering them active. Then, STAT transduces the signal to the nucleus by binding to the DNA, thus initiating the transcription of genes involved in immune cell division, activation, and recruitment. JAK inhibitors could therefore prevent cytokine storm associated with COVID-19. Nanoengineered therapeutics and vaccines might provide additional benefits via potentiating and prolonging the pharmacological effects of their loaded cargoes.

overview of the nanoengineering attempts for the design of therapeutics and vaccines for the management of COVID-19.

2.5 Antiviral therapy

Remdesivir (GS-5734) is a nucleoside analog. It is a prodrug of GS-441524, which resembles a viral nucleoside. It can inhibit the replication of multiple coronaviruses in respiratory epithelial cells by incorporating itself into the viral RNA with the aid of RNA-dependent RNA polymerase, thus producing defective RNA (Gordon et al., 2020). It has been used to treat the Ebola virus disease, and it is suggested for the management of COVID-19. It inhibited viral replication of clinical isolates of the SARS-CoV-2 virus in vitro. It also reduced viral load in animal models infected with MERS (de Wit et al., 2020; Sheahan et al., 2020). Results from clinical trials evaluating remdesivir in severe COVID-19 patients requiring no mechanical ventilation inferred no difference between a 5-days course and a 10-days course (Goldman et al., 2020). Because there was no placebo control in the study, the benefit of the therapy could not be determined. However, preliminary data from a placebo-controlled trial ($n = 1063$) in COVID-19 patients reported a lower mortality rate and shorter recovery time in patients treated with remdesivir versus placebo (Beigel et al., 2020). Remdesivir was evaluated in multiple clinical trials; a series of placebo-controlled double-blinded phase 3 trial ($n = 1062$) reported that remdesivir shortened the time to recovery and patients had less respiratory tract infection when compared with the placebo group (Beigel et al., 2020). Moreover, a *meta*-analysis was made to investigate remdesivir for the treatment of COVID-19 by obtaining databases from PubMed, EMBASE, Cochrane library, and ClinicalTrials.gov databases of three randomized trials ($n = 7334$) (from January 1, 2020 to November 5, 2020), it was found that there is very low certainty evidence of any association between remdesivir use and shorter recovery time; however, moderate certainty of evidence showed higher rates of patients recovery and discharge (Al-Abdouh et al., 2021). Remdesivir was the first to gain approval from the FDA for the treatment of COVID-19 (Food and Drug Administration, 2020). In an attempt to improve patient's compliance and dosage form convenience together with the reduction of personal contact, a self-injectable formulation of remdesivir was designed recently for the treatment of COVID-19. The formulation was fabricated using biodegradable and biocompatible poly(lactic-*co*-glycolic acid) (Patki et al., 2021).

Chloroquine and *hydroxychloroquine* are cheap oral prescription drugs with well-established clinical safety profiles that have been used for more than 70 years for the treatment of malaria and amebiasis, and for other antiinflammatory applications, such as the treatment of rheumatoid arthritis. Chloroquine, 4-aminoquinoline derivative, is rapidly and almost completely absorbed from the gastrointestinal tract following oral administration with a peak plasma concentration that is generally attained within 1−2 h. It is widely distributed in tissues, mostly excreted unchanged in the urine and partially metabolized in the liver. Its mechanism of action is not fully understood; however, it is believed to prevent viral entry, transport, and postentry events, and it possibly increases the pH of endosomes and lysosomes (Liu et al., 2020). The US Food and Drug Administration (FDA) has issued an emergency use authorization for chloroquine and hydroxychloroquine to treat patients hospitalized with COVID-19. Hydroxychloroquine and chloroquine have demonstrated in vitro activity against SARS-CoV-2 (Liu et al., 2020; Wang, Cao, et al., 2020; Wang, Hu, et al., 2020; Wang, Wang, et al., 2020). A combination of hydroxychloroquine and azithromycin had a synergistic effect in vitro on SARS-CoV-2 at concentrations compatible with that obtained in human lungs (Andreani et al., 2020). The use of hydroxychloroquine was increased recently in many countries as promising preliminary results regarding efficacy and safety in COVID-19 patients receiving a 10-days course were observed (Gao, Chen, et al., 2020; Gao, Tian, et al., 2020). In another bigger study ($n = 1061$), hydroxychloroquine and azithromycin combination were further investigated and good clinical outcomes and viral clearance were observed. In this study, it was concluded that the use of this combination was safe and resulted in a low fatality rate in patients when they were administered before COVID-19 complications occur (Million, 2020). In an attempt to further evaluate the clinical use of chloroquine, it was observed that high doses of chloroquine prolonged QT interval in the electrocardiography of patients; thus it is not recommended to use high doses in the management of COVID-19, especially in combination with azithromycin and oseltamivir and in old patients, due to safety concerns (Borba, 2020). In a multicenter, randomized, and controlled trial ($n = 250$), hydroxychloroquine did not improve therapeutic outcomes in mild-to-moderate COVID-19 patients at risk of disease progression (Vincent Dubée et al., 2021). However, in another single-center study

($n = 152$), it was found that hydroxychloroquine improved clinical condition in 91.4% of patients, and adverse effects were tolerable and were not associated with ventricular arrhythmia due to QT prolongation (Sogut et al., 2021). Despite these results, *meta*-analysis of multiple clinical trials reported no benefits with the use of hydroxychloroquine (Pathak et al., 2020). Yet more studies are being conducted on hydroxychloroquine, and future data availability will improve our knowledge about this drug (ClinicalTrials.gov: NCT04351620, NCT04329832, and NCT04429867).

Ivermectin is an antiparasitic drug that is approved by the FDA for the treatment of tropical diseases, including onchocerciasis, helminthiases, and scabies (Omura & Crump, 2014). There is an evidence from previous studies of the antiviral activity of ivermectin that it can inhibit RNA viruses such as Zika virus and Dengue virus (Barrows et al., 2016; Wagstaff et al., 2012). In an attempt to discover new treatments to overcome the rapidly upraising pandemic, in vitro studies were conducted and it was found that ivermectin reduced RNA replication of SARS-CoV-2 in vitro by 5000-fold within 48 h (Caly et al., 2020), and in vivo, in mice models, it demonstrated antiviral activity against mouse hepatitis virus, a type 2 family RNA coronavirus similar to SARS-CoV-2 (Arévalo et al., 2021). Clinically, ivermectin ($n = 24$) reduced COVID-19 symptoms and reduced viral load and antibody titers compared with controls (Chaccour, 2021). Furthermore, lower mortality was observed in COVID-19 patients treated with ivermectin, especially in those with severe pulmonary involvement (Rajter et al., 2021). Ivermectin is currently being tested in several clinical trials for the treatment of COVID-19 (NCT04425707, NCT04681053, NCT04723459, NCT04729140, and NCT04529525).

2.6 Lopinavir/ritonavir and Arbidol

Lopinavir and *ritonavir* are protease inhibitors that are used together in combination for the treatment of HIV infection. Results from a recent clinical trial ($n = 199$) evaluating either lopinavir or ritonavir treatment course (14 days) for severe COVID-19 demonstrated no benefits beyond the standard care (Cao et al., 2020). Lopinavir/ritonavir was further investigated in an ongoing trial "RECOVERY trial" ($n = 1919$), conducted across 176 hospitals in the United Kingdom. Released data showed no reduction in 28-days mortality, duration of hospital stay, and no risk of developing respiratory complications that might lead to respiratory intervention or death (Horby et al., 2020). Additionally, data from Solidarity trial included 11,330 adults; 2750 received remdesivir, 954 received hydroxychloroquine, 1411 received lopinavir (without interferon), 2063 received interferon (including 651 received a combination of interferon plus lopinavir), and 4088 received no treatment. Results indicated little or no difference between the test groups and control group with regard to mortality, need for mechanical ventilation, and duration of hospital stay (Pan et al., 2021). Besides, multiple clinical trials were further investigated on the use of these drugs in COVID-19 patients (ClinicalTrials.gov: NCT04346147, NCT04372628, and NCT04330690).

Arbidol is a broad-spectrum antiviral that is being used for the treatment of Influenza viral infections. It displayed antiviral activity against SARS-CoV-1 in vitro (Khamitov et al., 2008). It was indicated that arbidol can be beneficial in the treatment of COVID-19 patients and it demonstrated superiority to lopinavir/ritonavir with regard to its antiviral effects, although further studies in a greater number of subjects are needed (Zhu, Li, et al., 2020; Zhu, Lu, et al., 2020). In another retrospective cohort, combination therapy of lopinavir/ritonavir with arbidol was compared with lopinavir/ritonavir, and favorable clinical outcomes were observed for the arbidol combination therapy (Lisi et al., 2020). However, there were no differences observed in the phase IV trial ($n = 86$) for the management of mild/moderate COVID-19 regarding clinical outcomes and rate of conversion from positive to negative of the viral RNA between the studied groups, implying no benefit could be obtained with lopinavir/ritonavir or arbidol (Li et al., 2020). However, arbidol was further evaluated in a randomized trial ($n = 100$); two groups of patients were included; patients in one group received hydroxychloroquine followed by KALETRA (lopinavir/ritonavir) and patients in the other group received hydroxychloroquine followed by arbidol. Results indicated that arbidol improved patients' condition significantly when compared to KALETRA (lopinavir/ritonavir) in terms of improved peripheral oxygen saturation, duration of hospital stay, ICU admissions, and chest CT involvement together with improved laboratory investigations (Nojomi et al., 2020). A retrospective case series showed that arbidol resolved fever, decreased duration of hospital stay, and accelerated viral clearance from respiratory specimens especially in male patients (Gao, Chen, et al., 2020; Gao, Tian, et al., 2020). It is also being evaluated in multiple clinical trials (ClinicalTrials.gov: NCT04273763, NCT04286503, and NCT04260594).

Oseltamivir is a neuraminidase inhibitor that has been used in cases of MERS-CoV infection, and it is currently being evaluated clinically for efficacy and safety, for the management of COVID-19 (Borba, 2020). A recent study reported no benefit gained from administering oseltamivir to patients. It is being evaluated in several clinical trials in the management of COVID-19 (ClinicalTrials.gov: NCT04558463, NCT04516915, and NCT04338698).

2.7 Immune therapy

2.7.1 Convalescent plasma therapy

In a multicenter interventional study ($n = 368$); 135 COVID-19 patients received convalescent plasma, while 233 patients were controls. Moderate COVID-19 patients had a duration of 7 days to clinical improvement in the convalescent plasma group, while control group patients had a duration of 8 days ($P = .006$). Severe COVID-19 patients had a duration of 7 days to clinical improvement in the convalescent plasma group, versus 15.5 days in the control group ($P = .003$). Patients in the convalescent plasma group who were moderately ill had a significantly lower 30-day mortality rate than those from the control group. Moreover, after convalescent plasma transfusion, oxygen saturation improved within 3 days and lymphocyte counts increased on day 7 and day 14 in moderate COVID-19 patients and on day 11 and day 14 in severe COVID-19 patients. No adverse effects associated with convalescent plasma were reported in the study. Results showed possible benefits in reducing recovery time and rate in COVID-19 patients (Patki et al., 2021).

2.8 Tocilizumab

It is a recombinant humanized monoclonal antibody that blocks IL-6 receptors. It reduces cytokines production and acute-phase protein production. Its use has the potential to alleviate the hyperimmune state frequently reported in COVID-19 patients. Some cases reported improvement in clinical outcomes in patients with severe COVID-19 pneumonia who received anti-IL 6 (Cellina et al., 2020; Michot et al., 2020). Several retrospective cohorts found that the administration of tocilizumab reduced fever and the need for oxygen support and mechanical ventilation and led to an improvement in lung clinical presentation (Borku Uysal et al., 2020; Chilimuri et al., 2021; Guaraldi, 2020; Huang et al., 2021). However, data from recently conducted trial NCT04372186 ($n = 389$), which evaluated tocilizumab on COVID-19 patients with pneumonia versus placebo reported that tocilizumab reduced the risk of progressing to the need for mechanical ventilation, but it did not improve survival (Salama et al., 2021). In another study ($n = 452$), the tocilizumab patient's group showed no significant improvement in the clinical status or lower mortality of the COVID-19 patients than the placebo at 28 days (Rosas et al., 2021). Tocilizumab is currently being evaluated in several trials; alone (NCT04479358, NCT04435717) and in combination with remdesivir (NCT04409262) and with heparin in the HEPAMAP study (NCT04600141).

2.9 Bamlanivimab (LY3819253 or LY-CoV555) and Etesevimab (LY3832479 or LY-CoV016)

Bamlanivimab and Etesevimab are recombinant monoclonal antibodies that were isolated from SARS-CoV-2 patients and were further investigated for their efficacy against the virus (Jones et al., 2020). It was observed that they can bind to the S protein of the SARS-CoV-2 (Shi et al., 2020). Bamlanivimab was approved by the FDA for the treatment of mild–moderate COVID-19. They were investigated in the BLAZE-1 study phase 2/3 at 49 US centers ($N = 613$). The study groups included bamlanivimab alone, combination of bamlanivimab plus etesevimab, and placebo. Data showed a significant reduction in viral load in the drug combination group (bamlanivimab and etesevimab) when compared to placebo while no significant difference was observed in the viral load in bamlanivimab monotherapy group (Gottlieb et al., 2021). Currently, they are being tested in some trials (ClinicalTrials.gov: NCT04656691, NCT04796402, and NCT04701658).

2.10 Casirivimab (previously REGN10933) and imdevimab (previously REGN10987)

Casirivimab (previously REGN10933) and imdevimab (previously REGN10987) are recombinant human monoclonal antibodies. They bind to S proteins of SARS-CoV-2 and prevent its binding to ACE receptors (Pallotta et al., 2021). They are authorized for an emergency use for the management of mild-to-moderate COVID-19 cases who are at high risk of progressing to a severe state or who require hospitalization (FDA). In an attempt to prevent the appearance of resistant mutants of the SARS-CoV-2, a combination of two monoclonal antibodies casirivimab plus imdevimab were investigated in phase 1–3 trial ($n = 275$) and was assigned to a group of COVID-19 patients versus control group. Released results implied that the antibody combination is beneficial as it reduced viral load, especially in patients who had their immune response not yet elicited or who had a high baseline viral load (Weinreich et al., 2021). However, in a multicenter phase 3 trial (ACTIV-3), bamlanivimab, when given in combination with remdesivir, no benefit was reported in hospitalized COVID-19 patients who had no end-organ failure (Lundgren et al., 2021).

2.11 JAK inhibitors

JAK inhibitors are protein *kinases* that transduce cytokine-mediated signals via the *JAK*-STAT pathway including IL-6 and interferon-γ receptor signaling. They include *baricitinib*, *fedratinib*, and *ruxolitinib*, which are approved for rheumatoid arthritis, myelofibrosis, and psoriasis, respectively (Baricitinib for rheumatoid arthritis, 2019; Mesa, 2010; Mullally et al., 2020).

2.12 Baricitinib

Baricitinib is a JAK inhibitor that is selective for JAK1 and JAK2 and is FDA approved for the treatment of rheumatoid arthritis (Baricitinib, Olumiant, n.d.). Baricitinib received emergency use authorization from the FDA for treatment of COVID-19 (Fact Sheet for Healthcare Providers EUA for baricitinib, n.d.). It prevents inflammation by the inhibition of JAK1 and JAK2 in a pathway that involves STAT, in a dose-dependent manner, thus inhibiting subsequent proinflammatory signal of IL 6 in the immune cells (McInnes et al., 2019). Furthermore, an evidence of antiviral activity against SARS-CoV-2 was found, as it could prevent viral entry into the host lung cells. Also, in another study on macaques infected with SARS-CoV-2, it was found that baricitinib reduced inflammation in the lung and neutrophile recruitment and resulted in a reduction of macrophage-derived cytokines and chemokines production and decreased immune activation, thus limiting lung pathology (Hoang et al., 2021). Currently, it is being investigated in several clinical trials (NCT04421027, NCT04693026, and NCT04373044). A multicenter ACTT-2 trial ($n = 1033$) was conducted to evaluate baricitinib in combination with remdesivir for the treatment of moderate/severe

COVID-19 patients. Results demonstrated a median time to recovery of 7 and 8 days in the drug group and control group, respectively. Patients receiving high-flow oxygen or noninvasive ventilation had shorter recovery time in the tested group than the control group (10 vs 18 days). The 28-day mortality was 5.1% in the drug group and 7.8% in the control group. Moreover, patients from the tested group had less serious adverse events than those from the control group, thus implying the benefit that can be obtained from using this drug combination for hospitalized COVID-19 patients (Kalil et al., 2021).

2.13 Ruxolitinib

It is a JAK inhibitor that is used to manage myelofibrosis, policytemia vera, and hemophagocytic lymphohistiocytosis (Gálvez Acosta & Javalera Rincón, 2020; Hansen et al., 2021; Wang, Cao, et al., 2020; Wang, Hu, et al., 2020; Wang, Wang, et al., 2020). When tested in combination with steroids in a randomized clinical study versus placebo for the treatment of COVID-19, ruxolitinib significantly shortened recovery time in the treated group in contrast to that observed in the placebo group and no serious adverse events were encountered while using steroids nor ruxolitinib (D'Alessio et al., 2021). Data from another multicenter study ($n = 43$) conducted on severe COVID-19 patients reported promising results; patients had a numerically shorter time to clinical improvement. Significant chest computed tomography improvement and a faster recovery from lymphopenia were observed, and no serious adverse events were encountered with ruxolitinib. These data were enough to pursue further investigations (NCT04359290, NCT04355793, and NCT04377620).

2.14 Jakotinib

Jakotinib is another JAK inhibitor that is being tested in multiple clinical trials for various indications. JAK inhibitors could therefore prevent cytokine storm associated with COVID-19 (Felsenstein et al., 2020). However, JAK and STAT regulate interferon-controlled genes, thus blocking JAK-STAT will compromise interferon antiviral effects. Hence, their therapeutic use should be thoroughly evaluated in the management of COVID-19, and their potential therapeutic outcomes need to be weighed against possible adverse events (Favalli et al., 2020). Jakotinib and ruxolitinib were investigated for the management of COVID-19 in China (ChiCTR2000030170 and ChiCTR2000029580, respectively).

2.15 Vaccines

Vaccine development is crucial to control the spread of the disease among populations. A common strategy to control the rapid spreading nature of the virus is to establish herd immunity among populations, which is successfully reached when slightly <80% of the population becomes immune to SARS-CoV-2 (Fine et al., 2011). This can only be established if either a large population gets infected with the virus that does not seem to be the best scenario or by successfully immunizing this population with an effective vaccine. The fact that there is no country has reached herd immunity yet, and the strict social distancing when being removed, a second wave of the virus will most likely take place (Kamps & Hoffmann, 2020). Since COVID-19 crisis, there have been multiple global attempts to develop a vaccine for the novel coronavirus to place a hold on this uprising event. Vaccines are biomaterials designed to stimulate the host immune response against a specific pathogen, mainly an antigen-specific antibody response. There are several types of vaccines including living attenuated, inactivated vaccines, conjugate vaccines (weak and strong antigen conjugated together), subunit vaccines (fragment of the infectious agent), and recombinant vaccines (Vetter et al., 2018). Recombinant vaccines are synthesized with aid of a live viral or bacterial vector that is genetically engineered to express a specific antigen. Classic vaccines are derived from the causative microorganism. It could be whole living attenuated or inactivated vaccines. Synthetic vaccines are made up of synthetic peptide or polysaccharide antigens that are synthesized with the aid of recombinant genetic engineering technology (genes from two different species are inserted into a host organism to produce a specific bioproduct). They are considered to be safer than traditional vaccines. A balance between the safety and immunogenicity of the vaccine is important to maintain optimized immunization. Subunit vaccines are relatively safer than traditional vaccines; however, they are weakly immunogenic. Antigen nanoparticle vaccines might provide balanced immunogenicity and safety, which will be described later (*vide infra*) (López-Sagaseta et al., 2016). The S protein is an important candidate for vaccine development against coronavirus due to the crucial role of S protein in receptor attachment, membrane fusion, and cellular entry (Li et al., 2019). The S protein was used as a target for the design of mRNA, DNA, recombinant protein vaccines, and viral vector vaccines, for the SARS-CoV-2. In contrast, the whole virion was used to develop live attenuated vaccines and inactivated vaccines. Even though some immunization could be attained, previous studies have demonstrated that the whole inactivated SARS-CoV-1 vaccine results in pulmonary immunopathology and eosinophilic proinflammatory pulmonary response in vaccinated animals. Hence, recent efforts are being directed to other alternatives (Bolles et al., 2011; Lin et al., 2007; Spruth et al., 2006; Tseng et al., 2012).

2.16 Nanoengineered therapeutics and vaccines in development for management of COVID-19

2.16.1 Nanoengineered therapeutics

Several antivirals are being investigated for the treatment of COVID-19. Along the course of the investigation, many challenges regarding undesirable side effects, pharmacokinetic limitations, and pharmacodynamic issues are encountered. Nanoengineering constructs for encapsulation of these drugs could overcome the current challenges by enhancing cellular uptake of drugs, limiting undesirable side effects by controlling their bionavigation inside the body and reducing the dose needed to provide the desirable therapeutic effects. The ability to administer multiple drugs in the same vehicle can be also exploited for potential synergistic effects. Cellular uptake of nanoparticles encapsulating antivirals can be boosted by conjugating targeting moieties onto the surfaces of nanoparticles, which promote binding to cellular receptors and internalization, or by using specific polymer types that have an affinity to the target cells (Yang et al., 2002). Moreover, biodistribution can further be controlled with the aid of stimuli-responsive nanostructures. Pathological features describing a specific disease type can be exploited in the favor of nanoplatform design. For example, inflammation created during the course of infections leads to upregulation of intercellular adhesion molecule-1 (ICAM-1), which in turn increases the permeability of endothelial cells (Frank & Lisanti, 2008). In an attempt to exploit this phenomenon, γ3 peptide, which has a specific binding affinity to ICAM-1, was conjugated onto the surface of sparfloxacin- and tacrolimus-loaded poly(lactide-*co*-glycolide) nanoparticles, resulting in higher accumulation of nanoparticles in lungs (Yang et al., 2020). In COVID-19, the hyperimmune state can be exploited to control the bionavigation of nanoparticles inside the host body toward diseased areas, thus decreasing undesired accumulation in other tissues and consequently adverse events can be limited. In a previous study, endocytosis by hepatitis C virus-infected huh7.5 cells and its impact on cellular uptake of nanoparticles were studied, with the aid of confocal microscopy and flow cytometry. It was found that transfected cells had a higher accumulation of nanoparticles than nontransfected cells; thus it was concluded that viral transfection affected cellular uptake.

Physicochemical features of nanoparticles as surface charge, type of polymer, and protein corona formation also played a role in increasing cellular uptake of nanoparticles (Abo-zeid et al., 2018). Previous literature investigated the effect of size and charge on the cellular internalization by multiple lung cells, in an attempt to evaluate the impact of size and surface charge on the cellular uptake of nanoparticles by primary human alveolar type 1 (AT2) and primary human alveolar type 2 (AT2) cells. It was observed that negatively charged particles were taken up by 75% of the AT1 cells, while positively charged particles were taken up by $<55\%$ of these cells (Kemp et al., 2008). Effects of nanoparticle size together with nanoparticles surface modification were further investigated, and it was found that nanoparticles of sizes c. 50 nm interacted more with lung cells, while 100 nm particles interacted more with phagocytic cells. Latex polystyrene nanoparticles of size c. 50 nm were taken up passively by human alveolar epithelial type I-like cells (TT1), while those particles featuring size range 100 nm were taken up via receptor-mediated endocytosis. Also, it was found that amine-surface modified nanoparticles (ANP) were taken up more rapidly than carboxyl-surface modified nanoparticles and unmodified polystyrene nanoparticles (UNP), unlike TT1 cells that internalized the three types of nanoparticles. Primary human alveolar type 2 (AT2) cells internalized ANP only (Kemp et al., 2008).

Nanoengineering drugs have considerably aided in their delivery to their target sites together with improved pharmacokinetics and enhanced overall therapeutic outcomes. Drug release from nanoparticles can be altered to be immediate or sustained depending on the structural features of the nanoparticles. Specific sites in the body can be targeted by conjugating various ligands onto the surfaces of nanostructures that in turn increases drug amount reaching specific tissues, consequently, improving bioavailability, decreasing the dose administered, limiting adverse events, and reducing cost. Several examples exist in which nanomaterials offered several advantages for the delivery of drugs that possess antiviral activities against COVID-19. For instance, ribavirin is associated with severe hemolytic anemia due to massive accumulation in RBCs, which may require decreasing the ribavirin dose thus leading to a lower antiviral effect (Russmann et al., 2006). Ribavirin-loaded polymeric nanoparticles displayed lower accumulation in RBCs; thus therapeutic dose could be administered to preserve the antiviral activity of the drug (Abo-zeid & Garnett, 2020). When lopinavir was encapsulated inside nanoparticles, it possessed higher bioavailability as compared to free lopinavir (Ravi et al., 2014). Additionally, loading drugs in nanoengineered platforms allows for a dual administration of various drugs. Coadministration of ritonavir and lopinavir appeared to be quite beneficial as it lowers hepatic metabolism of lopinavir by cytochrome enzymes P450 3A4, thus improving bioavailability and reducing the administered dose. This dual administration was successfully approached by fabricating poly (lactide-*co*-glycolide) nanoparticles and loading both lopinavir and ritonavir into the nanoparticles (Abou-El-Naga et al., 2017). Nanostructures can be also employed to formulate poorly water-soluble drugs such as lopinavir. The poor water solubility of lopinavir results in low oral bioavailability. Loading of the drug into nanoparticles could enhance the overall solubility and could provide a dosage form that is more convenient for patients to improve patient compliance, especially with young children (the lopinavir formulation is currently available only in an adult form that should be extemporaneously divided into small doses for children) (Mahajan & Patil, 2020; Pham et al., 2016). It was reported that in situ self-assembly nanoparticles, based on oleic acid and D-α-tocopherol polyethylene glycol 1000 succinate (TPGS), successfully encapsulated lopinavir and ritonavir at significantly high encapsulation efficiency, improved their bioavailability, and provided adequate and stable plasma concentrations of drugs over 8 h. In addition, nanoparticles improved biodistribution via significantly increasing lopinavir concentrations by 2.8-fold in the liver, 5.1-fold in the kidney, 2.7-fold in the brain, 6.1-fold in the lymph nodes, and 3.4-fold in the spleen, as compared to free lopinavir/ritonavir combination (Pham et al., 2016). Lopinavir was incorporated also into vitamin E-TPGS micelle, which resulted in an enhanced aqueous solubility by 2.6-fold. When tested in vivo, an increase in oral bioavailability by 3.17 folds was found. The use of TPGS, as an encapsulating polymer, increased the stability of micelles, improved absorption of lopinavir, and inhibited P-glycoprotein, thus inhibiting efflux of lopinavir from cells (Mahajan & Patil, 2020; Tian & Mao, 2012). In another study, oseltamivir decorated onto the surface of silver nanoparticles has demonstrated higher antiviral activity against

H1N1 viral infection in vitro in Madin-Darby Canine Kidney cells and lower toxicity than free silver nanoparticles and free oseltamivir (Li et al., 2016).

Polyphosphate (PolyP) is a biologically derived polymer of endogenous anti-SARS-CoV-2 activity. The PolyP-encapsulated nanoparticles demonstrated strong interaction with RBD of the SARS-CoV-2 by binding to the arginine amino acid that is present at its surface, forming a covalent-like interaction (Woods & Ferré, 2005), which will subsequently prevent the interaction of the viral S proteins with ACE2 receptors present at the host cells surface in lung and in some other organs (Neufurth et al., 2020).

2.16.2 Nanoengineered vaccines

Nanocarriers serve as excellent platforms to stimulate immune response, both humoral and cell-mediated responses, against specific antigens. They can be fine-tuned to modulate immune response. Their size, shapes, surface charge, amphiphilicity, antigen display, antigen concentration greatly influence the extent and type of immune response elicited. Nanoparticles fabricated at sizes <200 nm have excellent lymphatic trafficking, can be easily accumulated at lymph nodes, engulfed by antigen-presenting cells, processed and presented to T cells, and enhance activation of B cells to secret specific antibodies. Free peptides are weakly immunogenic, owing to their inability to stimulate dendritic cell maturation, and they are eliminated rapidly from the host body. Hence, the incorporation of immunogenic peptides into appropriately designed nanomaterials triggers a greater immune response.

Viral antigen could either be adsorbed or conjugated onto the surface or encapsulated inside nanocarriers. Self-assembling protein nanoparticles are single protein monomers that are designed to self-assemble into nanoscale structures (Vetter et al., 2018). Synthetic virus-like particles (SVLP) are protein structures that resemble viruses in one or more antigens and are designed using recombinant technology. SVLP contain no genetic material and thus do not cause infection and they are nonreplicating (Negahdaripour et al., 2017). PEGylated nanoparticles showed the ability to improve lymphatic trafficking and biodistribution of the administered nanoconstructs (Zhuang et al., 2012). PEGylation also promotes mucoadhesion of nanovaccines administered to the nasal mucosa, facilitating their permeation, due to network formation between PEG chains and mucus from nasal mucosa (Huang et al., 2000; Sahlin & Peppas, 1997), and/or hydrogen bonds formation between the polymer and mucins (Lele & Hoffman, 2000; Yusuf et al., 2017).

There are many different shapes of nanoconstructs, each could be employed in a way to affect the properties of the nanovaccines, thus modifying the degree and duration of the elicited immune response. For example, utilizing nanofibers as vaccine platforms can enhance vaccine efficacy (Li et al., 2013; Si et al., 2018) and can allow for adjustable peptide display on their surfaces, which in turn, allow for improved peptide-specific immunization (Parlane et al., 2020). Dendrimers, repetitively branched polymeric constructs, have demonstrated intrinsic adjuvanticity that can be also utilized to boost the immune response (Lu et al., 2015). To enhance the immunogenicity of weakly immunogenic peptide antigens, dendrimers were constructed in star-shaped nanoparticles that allowed for modulating immunogen density and allowed for codelivery of T-helper antigens which also produced prolonged retention time at the injection site (Francica et al., 2019). Liposomes are phospholipid vesicles, with a structural mimicry to cell membranes. They can be used as vaccine delivery systems by loading them with viral antigens or via conjugation of antigens onto their surfaces. Moreover, liposomes possess intrinsic adjuvant activity, and they can stimulate dendritic cells by upregulating cytokines expression and activating ERK kinase (Yan et al., 2007). Over the past decades, liposomal adjuvanticity emerged to become frequently exploited as an important vaccine adjuvant-delivery system. Physicochemical features of liposomes that control the type, extent, and duration of the elicited immune response include surface charge, membrane fluidity, liposomal size, and whether antigens are loaded inside or conjugated/adsorbed onto their surfaces (Wang et al., 2019). The fluidity of membranes forming the liposomes depends primarily on the type of lipids. Longer chain lipids increase membrane rigidity while shorter ones decrease rigidity (Perrie et al., 2016). Incorporating cholesterol in liposomal structure showed to decrease membrane fluidity besides additional effects on particle size, morphology, and release of hydrophilic cargoes (Kaddah et al., 2018). Previous studies on the effect of membrane fluidity on the adjuvant activity of liposomes demonstrated that rigid membrane liposomes produced greater immune response, release of more antigens at the injection site, and higher stimulation of Th1 cells (Christensen et al., 2012). Additionally, it was previously observed that cationic liposomes trigger a higher immune response than that generated with either neutral or anionic liposomes (Davidsen et al., 2005). As well, cationic liposomes displayed an additional advantage, as they can deliver their cargos to the depot. Their surface positive charges allow for interaction with proteins from extracellular fluids leading to their aggregation, therefore, forming a depot at the administration site. This allows for retained antigen release and consequently prolonged immune response (Chatzikleanthous et al., 2020; Wilson et al., 2009).

Polymeric nanoparticles have been also frequently utilized for the design of nanovaccines, due to their intrinsic adjuvant properties (Zhang et al., 2018, 2019). Several polymers have been utilized in the fabrication process, such as chitosan (Bolhassani et al., 2014), poly(lactide-*co*-glycolide) (Yang et al., 2016), polyethylene glycol (Jain et al., 2010), and polypeptides (Xiang et al., 2018). Cationic nanoconstructs proved to improve cellular internalization and subsequent antigen delivery to cellular targets (Yue et al., 2011; Yusuf et al., 2017). Furthermore, complexation with nanoparticles could protect cargoes from enzymatic degradation, thus increasing whole vaccine stability, which is particularly important for mRNA and DNA-based vaccines due to their susceptibility to enzymatic degradation (Elsabahy et al., 2011). Utilization of nanostructures allows for optimizing antigen display in terms of antigen surface distribution and density, consequently, enhancing immune response (Francica et al., 2019) and improving B cell receptor cross-linking (Ingale et al., 2016). In addition to antigen display modulation, multiple antigens can be displayed simultaneously to receptors, and thus more effective stimulation of B cells can be attained (Kanekiyo et al., 2019).

Vaccine development can further be advanced by utilizing the relatively large loading capacity of nanostructures and fine-tuning of their structures and composition, thus encapsulating both antigens and additional adjuvants together. Furthermore, various immunomodulators can be incorporated into the formulation, either encapsulated inside the nanocarrier or conjugated onto the surface to further improve the effectiveness of the vaccine (Tallapaka et al., 2019). Moreover, nanoplatforms allow for controlled bionavigation with the aid of surface decorating moieties that improve cellular uptake via receptor-mediated endocytosis. The ability to control the release of the loaded cargoes allows control over the immune reactions generated. Controlling the release of antigens can be particularly useful for DNA vaccines due to the risk of insertional mutagenesis if high doses are administered. Hence, nanoplatforms can advance the overall safety of vaccines (Lu, 2020).

Upon introducing the vaccine into the host body, it enters the lymphatic system and becomes engulfed by antigen-presenting cells and presented to B cells. Then, B cells are stimulated to produce antigen-specific antibodies and IgM during an early primary immune response, and IgG is produced later and lasts longer than IgM. Multiple previous attempts to utilize nanomedical approaches in the design of coronavirus vaccines were frequently conducted for efficient immunization via the production of antigen-specific antibodies. For instance, homologous MERS spike protein nanoparticles and heterologous adenoviral vector/MERS-spike protein stimulated immunoglobulin IgG production. Simultaneous stimulation of Th1 and Th2 cells was only observed with heterologous adenoviral vector/MERS-spike protein, but not with spike protein nanoparticles alone, thus ultimately producing longer-lasting immunization. However, it was found that the host body secreted antibodies against the viral vector antigen, which led to decreasing antigen presentation to antigen-presenting cells, thus compromising the immune response elicited (Jung et al., 2018). Likewise, another study group developed two protein nanoparticle vaccines, one from S protein of SARS-CoV-1 and the other is from S protein of MERS. Both nanoparticles produced neutralizing antibodies against their respective antigens in mice. Two types of adjuvants, Alum and Matrix-M1, were evaluated in this study. Matrix-M1 induced immune response more effectively than Alum. However, no cross-immunity was observed, that is, each nanoparticle resulted in the immune response against the respective virus but not the other coronavirus (Coleman et al., 2014). Matrix-M1 is a saponin-based adjuvant that upon incorporation into the vaccine design increases vaccine immunogenicity and elicits both cellular and humoral immune responses while keeping a balance between Th1 and Th2 responses and eliciting cytotoxic T cell responses (Cox et al., 2011; Madhun et al., 2009; Magnusson et al., 2018; Pedersen et al., 2014). In an attempt to develop a vaccine against MERS-CoV, Matrix-M1 was combined with MERS-CoV S protein nanoparticles. Specific immunoglobulins were generated and the vaccine was able to stop replication in an in vivo mice model of MERS infection. The generated immunoglobulins were higher than those produced with MERS S nanoparticles alone, highlighting the immunomodulatory effect of Matrix-M1 in potentiating the immunogenicity of vaccines (Coleman et al., 2017). In another study, SVLP was fabricated by adsorbing S protein onto the surface of gold nanoparticles. SVLP showed an increased antigen delivery, lymphatic transport, lymph node localization, higher IgG production than the free S protein. The results imply the activation of other immune mechanisms such as complement activation, increased cellular internalization, and enhanced antigen presentation by antigen-presenting cells (Chen et al., 2016; Heesters et al., 2014; Reddy et al., 2006), thus highlighting the potential benefits nano-approaches could add up to the coronavirus vaccine design.

In agreement with previous literature, data from a recent study indicated that multivalent display of RBD on 2-protein components self-assembly nanoparticles (I53–50) boosts immune response elicited, the vaccine nanoparticles stimulated immune response and generated 10-fold higher levels of antibody titers than with that generated with perfusion-stabilized spike protein even when given at fivefold lower dose. Antibodies produced could react with several antigen epitopes of the RBD; therefore it is expected to stay effective despite the mutations that might occur. Furthermore, the vaccine produced a relatively lower binding: neutralizing ratio than that of convalescent serum (Walls, n.d.).

Moreover, multivalent antigen display can activate B cells to a greater extent than soluble antigens (Antanasijevic et al., 2020). Two-component self-assembly protein nanoparticles vaccine study reported relatively greater B cells activation than with that elicited with soluble antigens in vitro. In vivo, the vaccine nanoparticles elicited a humoral immune response with a relatively high level of antibody titers in macaques in addition to reduced viral infection and replication (Brouwer et al., 2021). Conformational design of nanoparticle vaccine platform for SARS-CoV-2 and HIV-1 viruses that constituted 1,2-Dioleoyl-sn-glycero-3-phosphocholine, *n*-(succinimidyloxy-glutaryl)-L-α-phosphatidylethanolamine, dioleoyl and monophosphoryl lipid A demonstrated an increased cellular uptake of antigens, antigen presentation, and enhanced dendritic cell activation. A high accumulation of antigen at lymph nodes was observed. When compared with soluble antigen proteins, a greater immune response was reported with regard to higher serum antibody titers against RBD of S receptor of the SARS-CoV-2 in mice (Park et al., 2021).

Multiple nanoplatforms can be employed in designing vaccines and therapeutics for the management of COVID-19 (Table 2.1), such as polymeric nanoparticles, inorganic nanoparticles, lipid-based nanostructures, virus-like nanoparticles, and self-assembled peptide nanoparticles (Keech et al., 2020; Press Release, 2021; Ramasamy et al., 2020).

Table 2.1 Nanoengineered vaccines and therapeutics in development for management of COVID-19.

Nanodevice	Type	Composition	Remarks	Reference
NVX-CoV2373	Vaccine	Solid lipid nanoparticle; comprised of ionizable lipid, SM-102, and 3 commercially available lipids, cholesterol, DSPC, and PEG2000-DMG	Results showed that the vaccine is safe and effective	ClinicalTrials.gov Identifier: NCT04368988
mRNA-1273 LNP	Vaccine	Recombinant peptide nanoparticle vaccine	Vaccine combined with Matrix-M1 as an adjuvant currently tested in phase 2	https://ir.novavax.com/news-releases/news-release-details/novavax-identifies-coronavirus-vaccine-candidate-accelerates (accessed on June 2021)
Ribavirin-loaded polymeric nanoparticles	Therapeutic	Polyglycerol-adipate (PGA) polymeric nanoparticles	Lower accumulation of ribavirin inside RBCs —lower toxicity	Abo-zeid et al. (2018)
Lopinavir-vitamin E-TPGS Micelle	Therapeutic	D-α-tocopherol polyethylene glycol 1000 succinate	Higher oral bioavailability than the free drug suspension	Mahajan and Patil (2020) and Pham et al. (2016).
Lopinavir-loaded polymeric nanoparticles	Therapeutic	Pullulan acetate polymer	Higher bioavailability than the free lopinavir	Ravi et al. (2014)

(Continued)

Table 2.1 (Continued)

Nanodevice	Type	Composition	Remarks	Reference
Lopinavir/ritonavir-loaded polymeric nanoparticles	Therapeutic	Poly(lactide-*co*-glycolide) copolymer	Higher bioavailability of lopinavir	Abou-El-Naga et al. (2017)
Lopinavir/ritonavir-loaded in situ self-assembly nanoparticles	Therapeutic	Oleic acid and D-α-tocopherol polyethylene glycol 1000 succinate	Enhanced oral bioavailability, stable therapeutic plasma concentrations, and improved biodistribution	Pham et al. (2016)
Oseltamivir modified silver nanoparticles	Therapeutic	Oseltamivir-modified silver nanoparticles	Higher antiviral activity and lower toxicity than the free drug and the unloaded silver nanoparticles	Li et al. (2016)

2.17 Current status and perspectives

Vaccines comprising *mRNA* are effective at eliciting immune responses, both innate and adaptive ones. Also, they are a relatively safe versatile approach in immunization, and their use neither involves the risk of insertional mutagenesis nor the risk of infection, although their instability necessitates their incorporation into a protecting platform (Pardi et al., 2018). They are safer than inactivated or protein-based vaccines because they are free from the risk of protein contamination or activation of an injected virus. Furthermore, mRNA vaccine possesses a superior advantage, which is on a large scale, and mRNA does not involve problems arising with the purification processes of viral proteins which are appreciated in saving time spent in standardization. In addition to the negative charge and the hydrophilic nature, the RNA cannot be taken up easily by the cells during in vivo conditions. Thus it requires highly efficient carriers such as nanoparticles. The lipid nanoparticle promotes mRNA vaccine stability and protects it from intracellular and extracellular degrading enzymes. In addition, the nanoparticles were biologically compatible and could aid in their cellular internalization (Elsabahy et al., 2011; Goswami et al., 2019; Samaridou et al., 2020).

Vaccines developed by Biontec and Pfizer are two mRNA encapsulated lipid nanoparticles vaccine candidates BNT162b1 and BNT162b2 that were tested in phase 1 trial ($n = 195$) in the United States and it involved multiple age groups (18–55 years and 65–85 years). Results elucidated showed similar serum antibody titers of the two vaccines and higher than that of convalescent individuals. Side effects were tolerable and were less with BNT162b2 than BNT162b1 (Walsh et al., 2020). The vaccine needs to be stored at −70°C, which can be very challenging when considering mass immunization. Data published from the phase 2 trial showed some early protection 12 days after the first dose, 7 days after the second dose, and 95% efficacy was reported (Polack et al., 2020).

University of Oxford together with AstraZeneca developed a *ChAdOx1 nCoV-19 vaccine*, which employs a chimpanzee adenoviral vector as a delivery vehicle that is being modified to be unable to replicate in the vaccinated host (Folegatti et al., 2019). The RNA encodes the S protein of the SARS-CoV2. The vaccine can be stored at regular refrigerator temperature that could be advantageous. Preclinical data in mice and in rhesus macaque models showed humoral and cellular immune responses. No pneumonia was observed in vaccinated rhesus macaques and no immune adverse events occurred (Doremalen, 2020). Upon testing this vaccine for safety, efficacy, and immunogenicity in two phase I/phase II clinical trials, one in the United Kingdom ($n = 1090$) and the other one in South Africa ($n = 2000$) (ClinicalTrials.gov: NCT04444674 and NCT04324606), similar neutralizing antibody titers between the study groups were observed, and T cell responses during the phase II trial ($n = 560$) were reported (Ramasamy et al., 2020). Currently, it is being evaluated in ongoing trials, phase II/III and phase III, respectively (ClinicalTrials.gov Identifier: NCT04400838 and NCT04516746).

The nanoengineered vaccine mRNA-1273 LNP showed promising preclinical and clinical results and is currently being tested in phase III trial ($n = 30{,}000$) (ClinicalTrials.gov: NCT04283461). The mRNA strand coding for the S protein of SARS-CoV-2 is encapsulated inside a lipid nanoparticle. It was developed by the National Institute of Allergy and Infectious Diseases of the National Institutes of Health together with Moderna, Inc. The vaccine requires −20°C to be stored, which could be available in developed countries and well-equipped health centers; however, in rural areas that are less equipped especially in developing countries, storage and transportation can be difficult.

Recombinant peptide nanoparticles vaccine (NVX-CoV2373) developed by Novavax, Inc. was tested in phase I clinical trial for safety and immunogenicity (ClinicalTrials.gov: NCT04368988), and results from phase I/II revealed that it is safe and potent as it elicited immune responses that exceeded levels in COVID-19 convalescent serum. Also, M-matrix is incorporated in the formulation as an adjuvant to boost immune response (Keech et al., 2020; Press Release, 2021).

iBioPharma, Inc. is developing two vaccines for COVID-19. *VLP* is a virus-like particle that is prepared by combining self-assembled proteins and SARS-CoV-2 antigen protein, and the resulting particles are further decorated with oligomannose monomers. The subunit vaccine is derived from SARS-CoV-2 S protein combined with lichenase booster molecule (LickM), a carrier protein molecule that is capable of augmenting the immune response generated by the vaccine.

CureVac Co. developed an mRNA vaccine that generated high levels of virus-neutralizing titers in animal models, and it is currently being tested in phase II/III trial (ClinicalTrials.gov Identifier: NCT04652102). Viral vector-based vaccines are also being developed. DNA vaccines are designed usually to encode specific antigens that can elicit immune responses against specific pathogens.

DNA vaccine for COVID-19 is being developed by Inovio Pharmaceuticals, Inc., which is called *INO-4800*. The vaccine encodes for the S protein of the SARS-CoV-2. Electroporationby a device called CELLECTRA produces a brief electrical pulse that makes small pores in the cell membrane to allow the transfection of plasmids. Preclinical data in animal models demonstrated that it is an effective vaccine in stimulating an immune response, both humoral and cell-mediated. It also produced neutralizing antibodies against the receptor-binding domain and results showed its effective neutralizing capacity of SARS-CoV-2, together with its competitive inhibition of the ACE2 receptors. The plasmid is stable at room temperature thus making it appropriate for mass immunization. Further investigations in bigger mammalian models and in human subjects are still needed (Smith et al., 2020).

Recombinant adenovirus type-5 (Ad5) vectored vaccine expressing S protein of SARS-CoV-2 was evaluated for safety and immunogenicity in phase I clinical trial ($n = 108$) (ClinicalTrials.gov: NCT04313127). Results published revealed that adverse events encountered with vaccine escalating dose were tolerable and no serious adverse effects were observed till 28 days postimmunization, and humoral and cellular immune responses were reported (Zhu, Li, et al., 2020; Zhu, Lu, et al., 2020).

The uprising global issue of COVID-19 motivated all parties to put in efforts to rapidly develop treatment and/or vaccines to limit the spread of the disease. Several recommendations and enormous efforts and endeavors have been proposed based on previous knowledge and expertise. In this chapter, the use of nanomedical approaches to develop potent therapeutics and vaccines against SARS-CoV-2 has been highlighted. Numerous structural and functional features of nanotherapeutics and nanovaccines have the potential to improve therapeutic efficacy and immunization strategies. However, it should be considered that to ultimately have an effective vaccine in the market available to mass populations worldwide, there are numerous stages of vaccine development. Vaccines might be also associated with immunopathologies, and thus investigating these candidate vaccines must be done with caution and all immune effects must be taken into consideration (Kamps & Hoffmann, 2020). For instance, the effect of immunizing ferrets with recombinant virus Ankara expressing S protein of SARS-CoV was studied, and severe hepatitis was demonstrated in the animal models (Kamps & Hoffmann, 2020; Weingartl et al., 2004). Furthermore, due to the complexity of the scale-up process, particularly with innovative and sophisticated technologies, nanoengineered therapeutics and vaccines may take up to several years to provide the market with sufficient amounts of safe yet efficient therapeutics and vaccines that can fulfill global demands.

Acknowledgment

M.E. and G.E. greatly acknowledge financial support from the Egyptian Science, Technology & Innovation Funding Authority (ID: 44534).

References

Abou-El-Naga, I. F., El Kerdany, E. D., Mady, R. F., Shalaby, T. I., & Zaytoun, E. M. (2017). The effect of lopinavir/ritonavir and lopinavir/ritonavir loaded PLGA nanoparticles on experimental toxoplasmosis. *Parasitology International*, *66*(6), 735–747. Available from https://doi.org/10.1016/j.parint.2017.08.007.

Abo-zeid, Y., Urbanowicz, R. A., Thomson, B. J., Irving, W. L., Tarr, A. W., & Garnett, M. C. (2018). Enhanced nanoparticle uptake into virus infected cells: Could nanoparticles be useful in antiviral therapy? *International Journal of Pharmaceutics*, *547*(1–2), 572–581. Available from https://doi.org/10.1016/j.ijpharm.2018.06.027.

Abo-zeid, Y., & Garnett, M. C. (2020). Polymer nanoparticle as a delivery system for ribavirin: Do nanoparticle avoid uptake by Red Blood Cells? *Journal of Drug Delivery Science and Technology*, *56*, 101552. Available from https://doi.org/10.1016/j.jddst.2020.101552.

Al-Abdouh, A., Bizanti, A., Barbarawi, M., Jabri, A., Kumar, A., Fashanu, O. E., Khan, S. U., Zhao, D., Antar, A. A. R., & Michos, E. D. (2021). Remdesivir for the treatment of COVID-19: A systematic review and *meta*-analysis of randomized controlled trials. *Contemporary Clinical Trials*, *101*. Available from https://doi.org/10.1016/j.cct.2021.106272.

Andreani, J., Le Bideau, M., Duflot, I., Jardot, P., Rolland, C., Boxberger, M., Wurtz, N., Rolain, J. M., Colson, P., La Scola, B., & Raoult, D. (2020). In vitro testing of combined hydroxychloroquine and azithromycin on SARS-CoV-2 shows synergistic effect. *Microbial Pathogenesis*, *145*. Available from https://doi.org/10.1016/j.micpath.2020.104228.

Antanasijevic, A., Ueda, G., Brouwer, P. J. M., Copps, J., Huang, D., Allen, J. D., Cottrell, C. A., Yasmeen, A., Sewall, L. M., Bontjer, I., Ketas, T. J., Turner, H. L., Berndsen, Z. T., Montefiori, D. C., Klasse, P. J., Crispin, M., Nemazee, D., Moore, J. P., Sanders, R. W., & Ward, A. B. (2020). Structural and functional evaluation of de novo-designed, two-component nanoparticle carriers for HIV Env trimer immunogens. *PLoS Pathogens*, *16*(8). Available from https://doi.org/10.1371/JOURNAL.PPAT.1008665.

Aust Prescr. (2019). *Baricitinib for rheumatoid arthritis*. Aust Prescr, 2019, **42**(1): p. 34–35.

Bani-Sadr, F., Hentzien, M., Pascard, M., Guyen, Y., Servettaz, A., Andreoletti, L., et al. (2020). *International Journal of Antimicrobial Agents*. https://doi.org/10.1016/j.ijantimicag.2020.106077.

Baricitinib Olumiant (n.d.). FDA, *Fact sheet for healthcare providers Emergency Use Authorization (EUA) of baricitinib*. From FDA. 2021. https://www.fda.gov/media/143823/download.

Baricitinib for rheumatoid arthritis. (2019). *Australian prescriber*, *42*, 34–35. Available from https://doi.org/10.18773/austprescr.2018.070.

Arévalo, A. P., Pagotto, R., Pórfido, J. L., Daghero, H., Segovia, M., Yamasaki, K., Varela, B., Hill, M., Verdes, J. M., Duhalde Vega, M., Bollati-Fogolín, M., & Crispo, M. (2021). Ivermectin reduces in vivo coronavirus infection in a mouse experimental model. *Scientific Reports, 11,* 1–12. Available from https://doi.org/10.1038/s41598-021-86679-0.

Barrows, N. J., Campos, R. K., Powell, S. T., Prasanth, K. R., Schott-Lerner, G., Soto-Acosta, R., Galarza-Muñoz, G., McGrath, E. L., Urrabaz-Garza, R., Gao, J., Wu, P., Menon, R., Saade, G., Fernandez-Salas, I., Rossi, S. L., Vasilakis, N., Routh, A., Bradrick, S. S., & Garcia-Blanco, M. A. (2016). A screen of FDA-approved drugs for inhibitors of zika virus infection. *Cell Host and Microbe, 20*(2), 259–270. Available from https://doi.org/10.1016/j.chom.2016.07.004.

Beigel, J. H., Tomashek, K. M., Dodd, L. E., Mehta, A. K., Zingman, B. S., Kalil, A. C., Hohmann, E., Chu, H. Y., Luetkemeyer, A., Kline, S., de Castilla, D., Finberg, R. W., Dierberg, K., Tapson, V., Hsieh, L., Patterson, T. F., Paredes, R., Sweeney, D. A., Short, W. R., Touloumi, G., Lye, D. C., Ohmagari, N., Oh, M., Ruiz-Palacios, G. M., Benfield, T., Fätkenheuer, G., Kortepeter, M. G., Atmar, R. L., Creech, C. B., Lundgren, J., Babiker, A. G., Pett, S., Neaton, J. D., Burgess, T. H., Bonnett, T., Green, M., Makowski, M., Osinusi, A., Nayak, S., & Lane, H. C. (2020). Remdesivir for the Treatment of Covid-19 — Final Report. *New England Journal of Medicine, 383,* 1813–1826. Available from https://doi.org/10.1056/NEJMoa2007764.

Bolhassani, A., Javanzad, S., Saleh, T., Hashemi, M., Aghasadeghi, M. R., & Sadat, S. M. (2014). Polymeric nanoparticles potent vectors for vaccine delivery targeting cancer and infectious diseases. *Human Vaccines and Immunotherapeutics, 10*(2), 321–332. Available from https://doi.org/10.4161/hv.26796.

Bolles, M., Deming, D., Long, K., Agnihothram, S., Whitmore, A., Ferris, M., Funkhouser, W., Gralinski, L., Totura, A., Heise, M., & Baric, R. S. (2011). A double-inactivated severe acute respiratory syndrome coronavirus vaccine provides incomplete protection in mice and induces increased eosinophilic proinflammatory pulmonary response upon challenge. *Journal of Virology, 85*(23), 12201–12215. Available from https://doi.org/10.1128/JVI.06048-11.

Borba, M. G. S. (2020). Effect of high vs low doses of chloroquine diphosphate as adjunctive therapy for patients hospitalized with severe acute respiratory syndrome coronavirus 2 (SARS-CoV-2) infection: A randomized clinical trial. *JAMA Network Open, 3* (4), e208857.

Borku Uysal, B., Ikitimur, H., Yavuzer, S., Ikitimur, B., Uysal, H., Islamoglu, M. S., Ozcan, E., Aktepe, E., Yavuzer, H., & Cengiz, M. (2020). Tocilizumab challenge: A series of cytokine storm therapy experiences in hospitalized COVID-19 pneumonia patients. *Journal of Medical Virology, 92*(11), 2648–2656. Available from https://doi.org/10.1002/jmv.26111.

Brouwer, P. J. M., Brinkkemper, M., Maisonnasse, P., Dereuddre-Bosquet, N., Grobben, M., Claireaux, M., de Gast, M., Marlin, R., Chesnais, V., Diry, S., Allen, J. D., Watanabe, Y., Giezen, J. M., Kerster, G., Turner, H. L., van der Straten, K., van der Linden, C. A., Aldon, Y., Naninck, T., & Sanders, R. W. (2021). Two-component spike nanoparticle vaccine protects macaques from SARS-CoV-2 infection. *Cell, 184* (5), 1188–1200. e19. Available from https://doi.org/10.1016/j.cell.2021.01.035.

Caly, L., Druce, J. D., Catton, M. G., Jans, D. A., & Wagstaff, K. M. (2020). The FDA-approved drug ivermectin inhibits the replication of SARS-CoV-2 in vitro. *Antiviral Research, 178.* Available from https://doi.org/10.1016/j.antiviral.2020.104787.

Cao, B., Wang, Y., Wen, D., Liu, W., Wang, J., Fan, G., Ruan, L., Song, B., Cai, Y., Wei, M., Li, X., Xia, J., Chen, N., Xiang, J., Yu, T., Bai, T., Xie, X., Zhang, L., Li, C., & Wang, C. (2020). A trial of lopinavir-ritonavir in adults hospitalized with severe covid-19. *New England Journal of Medicine, 382*(19), 1787–1799. Available from https://doi.org/10.1056/NEJMoa2001282.

Cellina, M., Orsi, M., Bombaci, F., Sala, M., Marino, P., & Oliva, G. (2020). Favorable changes of CT findings in a patient with COVID-19 pneumonia after treatment with tocilizumab. *Diagnostic and Interventional Imaging, 101*(5), 323–324. Available from https://doi.org/10.1016/j.diii.2020.03.010.

Chaccour, C. (2021). The effect of early treatment with ivermectin on viral load, symptoms and humoral response in patients with non-severe COVID-19: A pilot, double-blind, placebo-controlled, randomized clinical trial. *eClinicalMedicine, 32*, 100720.

Chan, J. F. W., Kok, K. H., Zhu, Z., Chu, H., To, K. K. W., Yuan, S., & Yuen, K. Y. (2020). Genomic characterization of the 2019 novel human-pathogenic coronavirus isolated from a patient with atypical pneumonia after visiting Wuhan. *Emerging Microbes and Infections, 9*(1), 221–236. Available from https://doi.org/10.1080/22221751.2020.1719902.

Chatzikleanthous, D., Schmidt, S. T., Buffi, G., Paciello, I., Cunliffe, R., Carboni, F., Romano, M. R., O'Hagan, D. T., D'Oro, U., Woods, S., Roberts, C. W., Perrie, Y., & Adamo, R. (2020). Design of a novel vaccine nanotechnology-based delivery system comprising CpGODN-protein conjugate anchored to liposomes. *Journal of Controlled Release, 323*, 125–137. Available from https://doi.org/10.1016/j.jconrel.2020.04.001.

Chen, H. W., Huang, C. Y., Lin, S. Y., Fang, Z. S., Hsu, C. H., Lin, J. C., Chen, Y. I., Yao, B. Y., & Hu, C. M. J. (2016). Synthetic virus-like particles prepared via protein corona formation enable effective vaccination in an avian model of coronavirus infection. *Biomaterials, 106*, 111–118. Available from https://doi.org/10.1016/j.biomaterials.2016.08.018.

Chilimuri, S., Sun, H., Alemam, A., Kang, K. S., Lao, P., Mantri, N., Schiller, L., Sharabun, M., Shehi, E., Tejada, J., Yugay, A., & Nayudu, S. K. (2021). Tocilizumab use in patients with moderate to severe COVID-19: A retrospective cohort study. *Journal of Clinical Pharmacy and Therapeutics, 46*(2), 440–446. Available from https://doi.org/10.1111/jcpt.13303.

Christensen, D., Henriksen-Lacey, M., Kamath, A. T., Lindenstrøm, T., Korsholm, K. S., Christensen, J. P., Rochat, A. F., Lambert, P. H., Andersen, P., Siegrist, C. A., Perrie, Y., & Agger, E. M. (2012). A cationic vaccine adjuvant based on a saturated quaternary ammonium lipid have different in vivo distribution kinetics and display a distinct CD4 T cell-inducing capacity compared to its unsaturated analog. *Journal of Controlled Release, 160*(3), 468–476. Available from https://doi.org/10.1016/j.jconrel.2012.03.016.

Chung, M., Bernheim, A., Mei, X., Zhang, N., Huang, M., Zeng, X., Cui, J., Xu, W., Yang, Y., Fayad, Z. A., Jacobi, A., Li, K., Li, S., & Shan, H. (2020). CT imaging features of 2019 novel coronavirus (2019-NCoV). *Radiology, 295*(1), 202–207. Available from https://doi.org/10.1148/radiol.2020200230.

Coleman, C. M., Liu, Y. V., Mu, H., Taylor, J. K., Massare, M., Flyer, D. C., Glenn, G. M., Smith, G. E., & Frieman, M. B. (2014). Purified coronavirus spike protein nanoparticles induce coronavirus neutralizing antibodies in mice. *Vaccine, 32*(26), 3169–3174. Available from https://doi.org/10.1016/j.vaccine.2014.04.016.

Coleman, C. M., Venkataraman, T., Liu, Y. V., Glenn, G. M., Smith, G. E., Flyer, D. C., & Frieman, M. B. (2017). MERS-CoV spike nanoparticles protect mice from MERS-CoV infection. *Vaccine, 35*(12), 1586–1589. Available from https://doi.org/10.1016/j.vaccine.2017.02.012.

Corman, V. M., Landt, O., Kaiser, M., Molenkamp, R., Meijer, A., Chu, D. K., et al. (2020). Detection of 2019 novel coronavirus (2019-nCoV) by real-time RT-PCR. *Eurosurveillance, 25*(3), 2000045.

Coronaviridae Study Group of the International Committee on Taxonomy of Viruses. (2020). The species Severe acute respiratory syndrome-related coronavirus: Classifying 2019-nCoV and naming it SARS-CoV-2. *Nature Microbiology, 5*, 536–544. Available from https://doi.org/10.1038/s41564-020-0695-z.

Coronavirus Disease (COVID-19) Pandemic. (2021). https://www.who.int/emergencies/diseases/novel-coronavirus-2019.

Covid-19 Treatment Guidelines. (2021). https://www.covid19treatmentguidelines.nih.gov/whats-new/-World Health Organization. (2020). Coronavirus disease (COVID-19): Dexamethasone. https://www.who.int/news-room/q-a-detail/q-a-dexamethasone-and-covid-19.

Cox, R. J., Pedersen, G., Madhun, A. S., Svindland, S., Sævik, M., Breakwell, L., Hoschler, K., Willemsen, M., Campitelli, L., Nøstbakken, J. K., Weverling, G. J., Klap, J., McCullough, K. C., Zambon, M., Kompier, R., & Sjursen, H. (2011). Evaluation of a virosomal H5N1 vaccine formulated with matrix MTM adjuvant in a phase I clinical trial. *Vaccine, 29*(45), 8049–8059. Available from https://doi.org/10.1016/j.vaccine.2011.08.042.

D'Alessio, A., Del Poggio, P., Bracchi, F., Cesana, G., Sertori, N., Di Mauro, D., Fargnoli, A., Motta, M., Giussani, C., Moro, P., Vitale, G., Giacomini, M., & Borra, G. (2021). Low-dose ruxolitinib plus steroid in severe SARS-CoV-2 pneumonia. *Leukemia, 35*(2), 635–638. Available from https://doi.org/10.1038/s41375-020-01087-z.

Davidsen, J., Rosenkrands, I., Christensen, D., Vangala, A., Kirby, D., Perrie, Y., Agger, E. M., & Andersen, P. (2005). Characterization of cationic liposomes based on dimethyldioctadecylammonium and synthetic cord factor from M. tuberculosis (trehalose 6,6′- dibehenate) – A novel adjuvant inducing both strong CMI and antibody responses. *Biochimica et Biophysica Acta – Biomembranes, 1718*(1–2), 22–31. Available from https://doi.org/10.1016/j.bbamem.2005.10.011.

de Haan, C. A. M., & Rottier, P. J. M. (2005). Molecular interactions in the assembly of coronaviruses. *Advances in Virus Research, 64*, 165–230. Available from https://doi.org/10.1016/S0065-3527(05)64006-7.

de Wit, E., Feldmann, F., Cronin, J., Jordan, R., Okumura, A., Thomas, T., Scott, D., Cihlar, T., & Feldmann, H. (2020). Prophylactic and therapeutic remdesivir (GS-5734) treatment in the rhesus macaque model of MERS-CoV infection. *Proceedings of the National Academy of Sciences of the United States of America, 117*(12), 6771–6776. Available from https://doi.org/10.1073/pnas.1922083117.

Doremalen. (2020). ChAdOx1 nCoV-19 vaccination prevents SARS-CoV-2 pneumonia in rhesus macaques. https://doi.org/10.1101/2020.05.13.093195.

Dubée, V., P.-M.R., Vielle, B., Parot-Schinkel, E., Blanchet, O., Darsonval, A., Lefeuvre, C., Abbara, C., Boucher, S., Devaud, E., Robineau, O., Rispal, P., Guimard, T., Anglejean, E., Diamantis, S., Custaud, M-A., Pellier, I., Mercat, A. (2021). Hydroxychloroquine in mild-to-moderate COVID-19: a placebo-controlled double blind trial. Clinical Microbiology and Infection, 27(8), 1124–1130. Available from https://doi.org/10.1016/j.cmi.2021.03.005.

Elsabahy, M., Nazarali, A., & Foldvari, M. (2011). Non-viral nucleic acid delivery: Key challenges and future directions. *Current Drug Delivery, 8*(3), 235–244. Available from https://doi.org/10.2174/156720111795256174.

Fact sheet for health care providers: Emergency use authorization (EUA) of REGEN-COVs (*casirivimab and imdevimab*). Available from: https://www.fda.gov/media/143893/download2020

FDA, Fact Sheet for Healthcare Providers EUA for baricitinib. Available at: https://www.fda.gov/media/143823/download.

Fadel, R., Morrison, A. R., Vahia, A., Smith, Z. R., Chaudhry, Z., Bhargava, P., Miller, J., Kenney, R. M., Alangaden, G., Ramesh, M. S., Nauriyal, V., Lakshmikanth, J.,

Abdul Hamed, A., Nadeem, O., Griebe, K., Johnson, J. M., Bradley, P., Uduman, J., Hegab, S., ... Scher, E. (2020). Early short-course corticosteroids in hospitalized patients with COVID-19. *Clinical Infectious Diseases, 71*(16), 2114–2120. Available from https://doi.org/10.1093/cid/ciaa601.

Favalli, E. G., Biggioggero, M., Maioli, G., & Caporali, R. (2020). Baricitinib for COVID-19: A suitable treatment? *The Lancet Infectious Diseases, 20*(9), 1012–1013. Available from https://doi.org/10.1016/S1473-3099(20)30262-0.

Felsenstein, S., Herbert, J. A., McNamara, P. S., & Hedrich, C. M. (2020). COVID-19: Immunology and treatment options. *Clinical Immunology, 215*. Available from https://doi.org/10.1016/j.clim.2020.108448.

Fine, P., Eames, K., & Heymann, D. L. (2011). \Herd immunity\: A rough guide. *Clinical Infectious Diseases, 52*(7), 911–916. Available from https://doi.org/10.1093/cid/cir007.

Folegatti, P. M., Bellamy, D., Roberts, R., Powlson, J., Edwards, N. J., Mair, C. F., Bowyer, G., Poulton, I., Mitton, C. H., Green, N., Berrie, E., Lawrie, A. M., Hill, A. V. S., Ewer, K. J., Hermon-Taylor, J., & Gilbert, S. C. (2019). Safety and immunogenicity of a novel recombinant simian adenovirus ChAdOx2 as a vectored vaccine. *Vaccines*, 7(2). Available from https://doi.org/10.3390/vaccines7020040.

Food and Drug Administration. (2020). https://www.fda.gov/news-events/press-announcements/fda-approves-first-treatment-covid-19.

Francica, J. R., Laga, R., Lynn, G. M., Mužíková, G., Androvič, L., Aussedat, B., Walkowicz, W. E., Padhan, K., Ramirez-Valdez, R. A., Parks, R., Schmidt, S. D., Flynn, B. J., Tsybovsky, Y., Stewart-Jones, G. B. E., Saunders, K. O., Baharom, F., Petrovas, C., Haynes, B. F., Seder, R. A., & Moon, J. J. (2019). Star nanoparticles delivering HIV-1 peptide minimal immunogens elicit near-native envelope antibody responses in nonhuman primates. *PLoS Biology, 17*(6), e3000328. Available from https://doi.org/10.1371/journal.pbio.3000328.

Frank, P. G., & Lisanti, M. P. (2008). ICAM-1: Role in inflammation and in the regulation of vascular permeability. *American Journal of Physiology – Heart and Circulatory Physiology, 295*(3), H926–H927. Available from https://doi.org/10.1152/ajpheart.00779.2008.

Gálvez Acosta, S., & Javalera Rincón, M. (2020). Ruxolitinib as first-line therapy in secondary hemophagocytic lymphohistiocytosis and HIV infection. *International Journal of Hematology, 112*(3), 418–421. Available from https://doi.org/10.1007/s12185-020-02882-1.

Gao, J., Tian, Z., & Yang, X. (2020). Breakthrough: Chloroquine phosphate has shown apparent efficacy in treatment of COVID-19 associated pneumonia in clinical studies. *BioScience Trends, 14*(1). Available from https://doi.org/10.5582/BST.2020.01047.

Gao, W., Chen, S., Wang, K., Chen, R., Guo, Q., Lu, J., Wu, X., He, Y., Yan, Q., Wang, S., Wang, F., Jin, L., Hua, J., & Li, Q. (2020). Clinical features and efficacy of antiviral drug, Arbidol in 220 nonemergency COVID-19 patients from East-West-Lake Shelter Hospital in Wuhan: A retrospective case series. *Virology Journal, 17*(1). Available from https://doi.org/10.1186/s12985-020-01428-5.

Goldman, J. D., Lye, D. C. B., Hui, D. S., Marks, K. M., Bruno, R., Montejano, R., Spinner, C. D., Galli, M., Ahn, M. Y., Nahass, R. G., Chen, Y. S., SenGupta, D., Hyland, R. H., Osinusi, A. O., Cao, H., Blair, C., Wei, X., Gaggar, A., Brainard, D. M., & Subramanian, A. (2020). Remdesivir for 5 or 10 days in patients with severe covid-19. *New England Journal of Medicine, 383*(19), 1827–1837. Available from https://doi.org/10.1056/NEJMoa2015301.

Gordon, C. J., Tchesnokov, E. P., Feng, J. Y., Porter, D. P., & Götte, M. (2020). The antiviral compound remdesivir potently inhibits RNAdependent RNA polymerase from Middle East respiratory syndrome coronavirus. *Journal of Biological Chemistry, 295* (15), 4773–4779. Available from https://doi.org/10.1074/jbc.AC120.013056.

Goswami, R., Chatzikleanthous, D., Lou, G., Giusti, F., Bonci, A., Taccone, M., Brazzoli, M., Gallorini, S., Ferlenghi, I., Berti, F., O'Hagan, D. T., Pergola, C., Baudner, B. C., & Adamo, R. (2019). Mannosylation of LNP results in improved potency for self-amplifying RNA (SAM) vaccines. *ACS Infectious Diseases, 5*(9), 1546–1558. Available from https://doi.org/10.1021/acsinfecdis.9b00084.

Gottlieb, R. L., Nirula, A., Chen, P., Boscia, J., Heller, B., Morris, J., Huhn, G., Cardona, J., Mocherla, B., Stosor, V., Shawa, I., Kumar, P., Adams, A. C., Van Naarden, J., Custer, K. L., Durante, M., Oakley, G., Schade, A. E., Holzer, T. R., & Skovronsky, D. M. (2021). Effect of bamlanivimab as monotherapy or in combination with etesevimab on viral load in patients with mild to moderate COVID-19: A randomized clinical trial. *JAMA – Journal of the American Medical Association, 325*(7), 632–644. Available from https://doi.org/10.1001/jama.2021.0202.

Grifoni, A., Weiskopf, D., Ramirez, S. I., Mateus, J., Dan, J. M., Moderbacher, C. R., Rawlings, S. A., Sutherland, A., Premkumar, L., Jadi, R. S., Marrama, D., de Silva, A. M., Frazier, A., Carlin, A. F., Greenbaum, J. A., Peters, B., Krammer, F., Smith, D. M., Crotty, S., & Sette, A. (2020). Targets of T Cell Responses to SARS-CoV-2 Coronavirus in Humans with COVID-19 Disease and Unexposed Individuals. *Cell, 181*, 1489–1501.e15. Available from https://doi.org/10.1016/j.cell.2020.05.015.

Guaraldi, G. (2020). Tocilizumab in patients with severe COVID-19: a retrospective cohort study. *The Lancet Rheumatology, 2*(8), E474–E484.

Hansen, S., Alduaij, W., Biggs, C. M., Belga, S., Luecke, K., Merkeley, H., & Chen, L. Y. C. (2021). Ruxolitinib as adjunctive therapy for secondary hemophagocytic lymphohistiocytosis: A case series. *European Journal of Haematology*. Available from https://doi.org/10.1111/ejh.13593.

Heesters, B. A., Myers, R. C., & Carroll, M. C. (2014). Follicular dendritic cells: Dynamic antigen libraries. *Nature Reviews Immunology, 14*(7), 495–504. Available from https://doi.org/10.1038/nri3689.

Hoang, T. N., Pino, M., Boddapati, A. K., Viox, E. G., Starke, C. E., Upadhyay, A. A., Gumber, S., Nekorchuk, M., Busman-Sahay, K., Strongin, Z., Harper, J. L., Tharp, G. K., Pellegrini, K. L., Kirejczyk, S., Zandi, K., Tao, S., Horton, T. R., Beagle, E. N., Mahar, E. A., & Paiardini, M. (2021). Baricitinib treatment resolves lower-airway macrophage inflammation and neutrophil recruitment in SARS-CoV-2-infected rhesus macaques. *Cell, 184*(2), 460–475.e21. Available from https://doi.org/10.1016/j.cell.2020.11.007.

Horby P. W., Mafham M., Bell J. L., Linsell L., Staplin N., Emberson J., Palfreeman A., Raw J., Elmahi E., Prudon B., Green C., Carley S., Chadwick D., Davies M., Wise M. P., Baillie J. K., Chappell L. C., Faust S. N., Jaki T., Jefferey K., Lim W. S., Montgomery A., Rowan K., Juszczak E., Haynes R., & Landray M. J. (2020). Lopinavir-ritonavir in patients admitted to hospital with COVID-19 (RECOVERY): a randomised, controlled, open-label, platform trial. *Lancet. 396*(10259), 1345–1352. Available from https://doi.org/10.1016/S0140-6736(20)32013-4.

Hoffmann, M., Kleine-Weber, H., Schroeder, S., Krüger, N., Herrler, T., Erichsen, S., Schiergens, T. S., Herrler, G., Wu, N.-H., Nitsche, A., Müller, M. A., Drosten, C., & Pöhlmann, S. (2020). SARS-CoV-2 Cell Entry Depends on ACE2 and TMPRSS2 and Is Blocked by a Clinically Proven Protease Inhibitor. *Cell, 181*, 271–280.e8. Available from https://doi.org/10.1016/j.cell.2020.02.052.

Huang, C., Wang, Y., Li, X., Ren, L., Zhao, J., Hu, Y., Zhang, L., Fan, G., Xu, J., Gu, X., Cheng, Z., Yu, T., Xia, J., Wei, Y., Wu, W., Xie, X., Yin, W., Li, H., Liu, M., & Cao, B. (2020). Clinical features of patients infected with 2019 novel coronavirus in Wuhan, China. *The Lancet, 395*(10223), 497–506. Available from https://doi.org/10.1016/S0140-6736(20)30183-5.

Huang, E., Isonaka, S., Yang, H., Salce, E., Rosales, E., & Jordan, S. C. (2021). Tocilizumab treatment in critically ill patients with COVID-19: A retrospective observational study. *International Journal of Infectious Diseases*, *105*, 245–251. Available from https://doi.org/10.1016/j.ijid.2021.02.057.

Huang, Y., Leobandung, W., Foss, A., & Peppas, N. A. (2000). Molecular aspects of muco- and bioadhesion: Tethered structures and site-specific surfaces. *Journal of Controlled Release*, *65*(1–2), 63–71. Available from https://doi.org/10.1016/S0168-3659(99)00233-3.

Ing, A. J., Cocks, C., & Green, J. P. (2020). COVID-19: In the footsteps of Ernest Shackleton. *Thorax*, *75*(8), 693–694. Available from https://doi.org/10.1136/thoraxjnl-2020-215091.

Ingale, J., Stano, A., Guenaga, J., Sharma, S. K., Nemazee, D., Zwick, M. B., & Wyatt, R. T. (2016). High-density array of well-ordered HIV-1 spikes on synthetic liposomal nanoparticles efficiently activate B cells. *Cell Reports*, *15*(9), 1986–1999. Available from https://doi.org/10.1016/j.celrep.2016.04.078.

Jain, A. K., Goyal, A. K., Mishra, N., Vaidya, B., Mangal, S., & Vyas, S. P. (2010). PEG-PLA-PEG block copolymeric nanoparticles for oral immunization against hepatitis B. *International Journal of Pharmaceutics*, *387*(1–2), 253–262. Available from https://doi.org/10.1016/j.ijpharm.2009.12.013.

Jones, B. E., Brown-Augsburger, P. L., Corbett, K. S., Westendorf, K., Davies, J., Cujec, T. P., Wiethoff, C. M., Blackbourne, J. L., Heinz, B. A., Foster, D., Higgs, R. E., Balasubramaniam, D., Wang, L., Bidshahri, R., Kraft, L., Hwang, Y., Žentelis, S., Jepson, K. R., Goya, R., Smith, M. A., Collins, D. W., Hinshaw, S. J., Tycho, S. A., Pellacani, D., Xiang, P., Muthuraman, K., Sobhanifar, S., Piper, M. H., Triana, F. J., Hendle, J., Pustilnik, A., Adams, A. C., Berens, S. J., Baric, R. S., Martinez, D. R., Cross, R. W., Geisbert, T. W., Borisevich, V., Abiona, O., Belli, H. M., de Vries, M., Mohamed, A., Dittmann, M., Samanovic, M., Mulligan, M.J., Goldsmith, J. A., Hsieh, C.-L., Johnson, N. V, Wrapp, D., McLellan, J. S., Barnhart, B. C., Graham, B. S., Mascola, J. R., Hansen, C. L., Falconer, E., 2020. LY-CoV555, a rapidly isolated potent neutralizing antibody, provides protection in a non-human primate model of SARS-CoV-2 infection. bioRxiv: the preprint server for biology. Available from https://doi.org/10.1101/2020.09.30.318972.

Jung, S. Y., Kang, K. W., Lee, E. Y., Seo, D. W., Kim, H. L., Kim, H., Kwon, T. W., Park, H. L., Kim, H., Lee, S. M., & Nam, J. H. (2018). Heterologous prime–boost vaccination with adenoviral vector and protein nanoparticles induces both Th1 and Th2 responses against Middle East respiratory syndrome coronavirus. *Vaccine*, *36*(24), 3468–3476. Available from https://doi.org/10.1016/j.vaccine.2018.04.082.

Kaddah, S., Khreich, N., Kaddah, F., Charcosset, C., & Greige-Gerges, H. (2018). Cholesterol modulates the liposome membrane fluidity and permeability for a hydrophilic molecule. *Food and Chemical Toxicology*, *113*, 40–48. Available from https://doi.org/10.1016/j.fct.2018.01.017.

Kalil, A. C., Patterson, T. F., Mehta, A. K., Tomashek, K. M., Wolfe, C. R., Ghazaryan, V., Marconi, V. C., Ruiz-Palacios, G. M., Hsieh, L., Kline, S., Tapson, V., Iovine, N. M., Jain, M. K., Sweeney, D. A., El Sahly, H. M., Branche, A. R., Pineda, J. R., Lye, D. C., Sandkovsky, U., … Beigel, J. H. (2021). Baricitinib plus remdesivir for hospitalized adults with Covid-19. *New England Journal of Medicine*, *384*(9), 795–807. Available from https://doi.org/10.1056/NEJMoa2031994.

Kamps, B. S., & Hoffmann, C. (2020). *COVID Reference* (4th ed). Steinhäuser Verlag.

Kanekiyo, M., Joyce, M. G., Gillespie, R. A., Gallagher, J. R., Andrews, S. F., Yassine, H. M., Wheatley, A. K., Fisher, B. E., Ambrozak, D. R., Creanga, A., Leung, K., Yang, E. S., Boyoglu-Barnum, S., Georgiev, I. S., Tsybovsky, Y., Prabhakaran, M. S., Andersen, H., Kong, W. P., Baxa, U., & Graham, B. S. (2019). Mosaic nanoparticle display of diverse influenza virus hemagglutinins elicits broad B cell responses. *Nature Immunology, 20*(3), 362–372. Available from https://doi.org/10.1038/s41590-018-0305-x.

Keech, C., Albert, G., Cho, I., Robertson, A., Reed, P., Neal, S., Plested, J. S., Zhu, M., Cloney-Clark, S., Zhou, H., Smith, G., Patel, N., Frieman, M. B., Haupt, R. E., Logue, J., McGrath, M., Weston, S., Piedra, P. A., Desai, C., & Glenn, G. M. (2020). Phase 1–2 trial of a SARS-CoV-2 recombinant spike protein nanoparticle vaccine. *New England Journal of Medicine, 383*(24), 2320–2332. Available from https://doi.org/10.1056/NEJMoa2026920.

Kemp, S. J., Thorley, A. J., Gorelik, J., Seckl, M. J., O'Hare, M. J., Arcaro, A., Korchev, Y., Goldstraw, P., & Tetley, T. D. (2008). Immortalization of human alveolar epithelial cells to investigate nanoparticle uptake. *American Journal of Respiratory Cell and Molecular Biology, 39*(5), 591–597. Available from https://doi.org/10.1165/rcmb.2007-0334OC.

Khamitov, R. A., Loginova, S. Y., Shchukina, V. N., Borisevich, S. V., Maksimov, V. A., & Shuster, A. M. (2008). Antiviral activity of arbidol and its derivatives against the pathogen of severe acute respiratory syndrome in the cell cultures. *Voprosy Virusologii, 53*(4), 9–13. Available from https://virusjour.elpub.ru/jour/issue/archive.

Kuppalli, K., & Rasmussen, A. L. (2020). A glimpse into the eye of the COVID-19 cytokine storm. *EbioMedicine, 55*, 102789.

Lele, B. S., & Hoffman, A. S. (2000). Mucoadhesive drug carriers based on complexes of poly(acrylic acid) and PEGylated drugs having hydrolysable PEG-anhydride-drug linkages. *Journal of Controlled Release, 69*(2), 237–248. Available from https://doi.org/10.1016/S0168-3659(00)00303-5.

Li, X., Galliher-Beckley, A., Huang, H., Sun, X., & Shi, J. (2013). Peptide nanofiber hydrogel adjuvanted live virus vaccine enhances cross-protective immunity to porcine reproductive and respiratory syndrome virus. *Vaccine, 31*(41), 4508–4515. Available from https://doi.org/10.1016/j.vaccine.2013.07.080.

Li, Y. H., Hu, C. Y., Wu, N. P., Yao, H. P., & Li, L. J. (2019). Molecular characteristics, functions, and related pathogenicity of MERS-CoV proteins. *Engineering, 5*(5), 940–947. Available from https://doi.org/10.1016/j.eng.2018.11.035.

Li, Y., Lin, Z., Zhao, M., Xu, T., Wang, C., Hua, L., Wang, H., Xia, H., & Zhu, B. (2016). Silver nanoparticle based codelivery of oseltamivir to inhibit the activity of the H1N1 influenza virus through ROS-mediated signaling pathways. *ACS Applied Materials and Interfaces, 8*(37), 24385–24393. Available from https://doi.org/10.1021/acsami.6b06613.

Li, Y., Xie, Z., Lin, W., Cai, W., Wen, C., Guan, Y., Mo, X., Wang, J., Wang, Y., Peng, P., Chen, X., Hong, W., Xiao, G., Liu, J., Zhang, L., Hu, F., Li, F., Zhang, F., Deng, X., & Li, L. (2020). *Efficacy and safety of lopinavir/ritonavir or arbidol in adult patients with mild/moderate COVID-19: an exploratory randomized controlled trial, 1*(1), 105–113.e4. Available from https://doi.org/10.1016/j.medj.2020.04.001.

Lin, J. T., Zhang, J. S., Su, N., Xu, J. G., Wang, N., Chen, J. T., Chen, X., Liu, Y. X., Gao, H., Jia, Y. P., Liu, Y., Sun, R. H., Wang, X., Yu, D. Z., Hai, R., Gao, Q., Ning, Y., Wang, H. X., Li, M. C., & Dong, X. P. (2007). Safety and immunogenicity from a phase I trial of inactivated severe acute respiratory syndrome coronavirus vaccine. *Antiviral Therapy, 12*(7), 1107–1113.

Lisi, D., Chunna, L., Qi, Z., Xi, L., Xinghua, L., Haitang, Z., Zhongsi, H., & Jinyu, X. (2020). Arbidol combined with LPV/r vs LPV/r alone against Corona virus disease 2019: A retrospective cohort study. *Journal of Infection, 81*(1), e1–e5. Available from https://doi.org/10.1016/j.jinf.2020.03.002.

Liu, J., Cao, R., Xu, M., Wang, X., Zhang, H., Hu, H., Li, Y., Hu, Z., Zhong, W., & Wang, M. (2020). Hydroxychloroquine, a less toxic derivative of chloroquine, is effective in inhibiting SARS-CoV-2 infection in vitro. *Cell Discovery*, *6*(1). Available from https://doi.org/10.1038/s41421-020-0156-0.

López-Sagaseta, J., Malito, E., Rappuoli, R., & Bottomley, M. J. (2016). Self-assembling protein nanoparticles in the design of vaccines. *Computational and Structural Biotechnology Journal*, *14*, 58–68. Available from https://doi.org/10.1016/j.csbj.2015.11.001.

Lu, F., Mencia, A., Bi, L., Taylor, A., Yao, Y., & HogenEsch, H. (2015). Dendrimer-like alpha-d-glucan nanoparticles activate dendritic cells and are effective vaccine adjuvants. *Journal of Controlled Release*, *204*, 51–59. Available from https://doi.org/10.1016/j.jconrel.2015.03.002.

Lu, X., Chen, T., Wang, Y., Wang, J., & Yan, F. (2020). Adjuvant corticosteroid therapy for critically ill patients with COVID-19. *Critical Care*, *24*(1), 241.

Lu, Y. (2020). Engineering a "PEG-g-PEI/DNA nanoparticle-in- PLGA microsphere" hybrid controlled release system to enhance immunogenicity of DNA vaccine. *Material Science Engineering C Materials for Biological Application*, 106.

Lundgren, J. D., Grund, B., Barkauskas, C. E., Holland, T. L., Gottlieb, R. L., Sandkovsky, U., Brown, S. M., Knowlton, K. U., Self, W. H., Files, D. C., Jain, M. K., Benfield, T., Bowdish, M. E., Leshnower, B. G., Baker, J. V., Jensen, J. U., Gardner, E. M., Ginde, A. A., Harris, E. S., & Neaton, J. D. (2021). A neutralizing monoclonal antibody for hospitalized patients with Covid-19. *New England Journal of Medicine*, *384*(10), 905–914. Available from https://doi.org/10.1056/NEJMoa2033130.

Madhun, A. S., Haaheim, L. R., Nilsen, M. V., & Cox, R. J. (2009). Intramuscular Matrix-M-adjuvanted virosomal H5N1 vaccine induces high frequencies of multifunctional Th1 CD4 + cells and strong antibody responses in mice. *Vaccine*, *27*(52), 7367–7376. Available from https://doi.org/10.1016/j.vaccine.2009.09.044.

Magnusson, S. E., Altenburg, A. F., Bengtsson, K. L., Bosman, F., de Vries, R. D., Rimmelzwaan, G. F., & Stertman, L. (2018). Matrix-MTM adjuvant enhances immunogenicity of both protein- and modified vaccinia virus Ankara-based influenza vaccines in mice. *Immunologic Research*, *66*(2), 224–233. Available from https://doi.org/10.1007/s12026-018-8991-x.

Mahajan, H. S., & Patil, P. H. (2020). Central composite design-based optimization of lopinavir vitamin E-TPGS micelle: In vitro characterization and in vivo pharmacokinetic study. *Colloids and Surfaces B: Biointerfaces*, *194*, 111149.

McInnes, I. B., Byers, N. L., Higgs, R. E., Lee, J., Macias, W. L., Na, S., Ortmann, R. A., Rocha, G., Rooney, T. P., Wehrman, T., Zhang, X., Zuckerman, S. H., & Taylor, P. C. (2019). Comparison of baricitinib, upadacitinib, and tofacitinib mediated regulation of cytokine signaling in human leukocyte subpopulations. *Arthritis Research and Therapy*, *21*(1). Available from https://doi.org/10.1186/s13075-019-1964-1.

Mesa, R. A. (2010). Ruxolitinib, a selective JAK1 and JAK2 inhibitor for the treatment of myeloproliferative neoplasms and psoriasis. *IDrugs*, *13*(6), 394–403.

Michot, J. M., Albiges, L., Chaput, N., Saada, V., Pommeret, F., Griscelli, F., Balleyguier, C., Besse, B., Marabelle, A., Netzer, F., Merad, M., Robert, C., Barlesi, F., Gachot, B., & Stoclin, A. (2020). Tocilizumab, an anti-IL-6 receptor antibody, to treat COVID-19-related respiratory failure: a case report. *Annals of Oncology*, *31*(7), 961–964. Available from https://doi.org/10.1016/j.annonc.2020.03.300.

Million, M. (2020). Full-length title: Early treatment of COVID-19 patients with hydroxychloroquine and azithromycin: A retrospective analysis of 1061 cases in Marseille, France. *Travel Medicine and Infectious Disease*, *35*, 101738.

Mullally, A., Hood, J., Harrison, C., & Mesa, R. (2020). Fedratinib in myelofibrosis. *Blood Advances, 4*(8), 1792–1800. Available from https://doi.org/10.1182/bloodadvances.2019000954.

Negahdaripour, M., Golkar, N., Hajighahramani, N., Kianpour, S., Nezafat, N., & Ghasemi, Y. (2017). Harnessing self-assembled peptide nanoparticles in epitope vaccine design. *Biotechnology Advances, 35*(5), 575–596. Available from https://doi.org/10.1016/j.biotechadv.2017.05.002.

Neufurth, M., Wang, X., Tolba, E., Lieberwirth, I., Wang, S., Schröder, H. C., & Müller, W. E. G. (2020). The inorganic polymer, polyphosphate, blocks binding of SARS-CoV-2 spike protein to ACE2 receptor at physiological concentrations. *Biochemical Pharmacology, 182*. Available from https://doi.org/10.1016/j.bcp.2020.114215.

Nojomi, M., Yassin, Z., Keyvani, H., Makiani, M. J., Roham, M., Laali, A., Dehghan, N., Navaei, M., & Ranjbar, M. (2020). Effect of Arbidol (Umifenovir) on COVID-19: A randomized controlled trial. *BMC Infectious Diseases, 20*(1). Available from https://doi.org/10.1186/s12879-020-05698-w.

Omura, S., & Crump, A. (2014). Ivermectin: Panacea for resource-poor communities? *Trends in Parasitology, 30*(9), 445–455. Available from https://doi.org/10.1016/j.pt.2014.07.005.

Pallotta, A. M., Kim, C. Y., Gordon, S. M., & Kim, A. (2021). Monoclonal antibodies for treating COVID-19. *Cleveland Clinic Journal of Medicine*. Available from https://doi.org/10.3949/ccjm.88a.ccc074.

Pan, H., Peto, R., Henao-Restrepo, A. M., Preziosi, M. P., Sathiyamoorthy, V., Karim, Q. A., Alejandria, M. M., García, C. H., Kieny, M. P., Malekzadeh, R., Murthy, S., Srinath Reddy, K., Periago, M. R., Hanna, P. A., Ader, F., Al-Bader, A. M., Alhasawi, A., Allum, E., Alotaibi, A., & Swaminathan, S. (2021). Repurposed antiviral drugs for COVID-19—InteriM WHO solidarity trial results. *New England Journal of Medicine, 384*(6), 497–511. Available from https://doi.org/10.1056/NEJMoa2023184.

Pardi, N., Hogan, M. J., Porter, F. W., & Weissman, D. (2018). mRNA vaccines-a new era in vaccinology. *Nature Reviews Drug Discovery, 17*(4), 261–279. Available from https://doi.org/10.1038/nrd.2017.243.

Park, K. S., Bazzill, J. D., Son, S., Nam, J., Shin, S. W., Ochyl, L. J., Stuckey, J. A., Meagher, J. L., Chang, L., Song, J., Montefiori, D. C., LaBranche, C. C., Smith, J. L., Xu, J., & Moon, J. J. (2021). Lipid-based vaccine nanoparticles for induction of humoral immune responses against HIV-1 and SARS-CoV-2. *Journal of Controlled Release, 330*, 529–539. Available from https://doi.org/10.1016/j.jconrel.2020.12.031.

Parlane, N. A., Wedlock, D. N., Han, J. H., & Park, J. H. (2020). Heterologous peptide display on chromatin nanofibers: A new strategy for peptide vaccines. *Biochemical and Biophysical Research Communications, 524*(4), 825–831. Available from https://doi.org/10.1016/j.bbrc.2020.02.004.

Pathak, D. S. K., Salunke, D. A. A., Thivari, D. P., Pandey, A., Nandy, D. K., Harish, V. K., Ratna, D., Pandey, D. S., Chawla, D. J., Mujawar, D. J., Dhanwate, D. A., & Menon, D. V. (2020). No benefit of hydroxychloroquine in COVID-19: Results of systematic review and *meta*-analysis of randomized controlled trials. *Diabetes and Metabolic Syndrome: Clinical Research and Reviews, 14*(6), 1673–1680. Available from https://doi.org/10.1016/j.dsx.2020.08.033.

Patki, M., Palekar, S., Reznik, S., & Patel, K. (2021). Self-injectable extended release formulation of Remdesivir (SelfExRem): A potential formulation alternative for COVID-19 treatment. *International Journal of Pharmaceutics, 597*. Available from https://doi.org/10.1016/j.ijpharm.2021.120329.

Pedersen, G. K., Sjursen, H., Nøstbakken, J. K., Jul-Larsen, Å., Hoschler, K., & Cox, R. J. (2014). Matrix MTM adjuvanted virosomal H5N1 vaccine induces balanced Th1/Th2 CD4 + T cell responses in man. *Human Vaccines and Immunotherapeutics, 10* (8), 2408–2416. Available from https://doi.org/10.4161/hv.29583.

Perrie, Y., Crofts, F., Devitt, A., Griffiths, H. R., Kastner, E., & Nadella, V. (2016). Designing liposomal adjuvants for the next generation of vaccines. *Advanced Drug Delivery Reviews, 99*, 85–96. Available from https://doi.org/10.1016/j.addr.2015.11.005.

Pham, K., Li, D., Guo, S., Penzak, S., & Dong, X. (2016). Development and in vivo evaluation of child-friendly lopinavir/ritonavir pediatric granules utilizing novel in situ self-assembly nanoparticles. *Journal of Controlled Release, 226*, 88–97. Available from https://doi.org/10.1016/j.jconrel.2016.02.001.

Polack, F. P., Thomas, S. J., Kitchin, N., Absalon, J., Gurtman, A., Lockhart, S., Perez, J. L., Marc, G. P., Moreira, E. D., Zerbini, C., Bailey, R., Swanson, K. A., Roychoudhury, S., Koury, K., Li, P., Kalina, W. V., Cooper, D., Frenck, R. W., Hammitt, L. L., & Gruber, W. C. (2020). Safety and efficacy of the BNT162b2 mRNA Covid-19 vaccine. *New England Journal of Medicine, 383*(27), 2603–2615. Available from https://doi.org/10.1056/NEJMoa2034577.

Press Release. (2021). https://ir.novavax.com/news-releases/news-release-details/novavax-identifies-coronavirus-vaccine-candidate-accelerates.

Rajter, J. C., Sherman, M. S., Fatteh, N., Vogel, F., Sacks, J., & Rajter, J. J. (2021). Use of ivermectin is associated with lower mortality in hospitalized patients with coronavirus disease 2019: The ivermectin in COVID nineteen study. *Chest, 159*(1), 85–92. Available from https://doi.org/10.1016/j.chest.2020.10.009.

Ramasamy, M. N., Minassian, A. M., Ewer, K. J., Flaxman, A. L., Folegatti, P. M., Owens, D. R., Voysey, M., Aley, P. K., Angus, B., Babbage, G., Belij-Rammerstorfer, S., Berry, L., Bibi, S., Bittaye, M., Cathie, K., Chappell, H., Charlton, S., Cicconi, P., Clutterbuck, E. A., & Zizi, D. (2020). Safety and immunogenicity of ChAdOx1 nCoV-19 vaccine administered in a prime-boost regimen in young and old adults (COV002): A single-blind, randomised, controlled, phase 2/3 trial. *The Lancet, 396*(10267), 1979–1993. Available from https://doi.org/10.1016/S0140-6736(20)32466-1.

Ravi, P. R., Vats, R., Balija, J., Adapa, S. P. N., & Aditya, N. (2014). Modified pullulan nanoparticles for oral delivery of lopinavir: Formulation and pharmacokinetic evaluation. *Carbohydrate Polymers, 110*, 320–328. Available from https://doi.org/10.1016/j.carbpol.2014.03.099.

Reddy, S. T., Berk, D. A., Jain, R. K., & Swartz, M. A. (2006). A sensitive in vivo model for quantifying interstitial convective transport of injected macromolecules and nanoparticles. *Journal of Applied Physiology, 101*(4), 1162–1169. Available from https://doi.org/10.1152/japplphysiol.00389.2006.

Rodriguez-Morales, A. J., Cardona-Ospina, J. A., Gutierrez-Ocampo, E., Villamizar-Pena, R., Holguin-Rivera, Y., Escalera-Antezana, J. P., et al. (2020). Clinical, laboratory and imaging features of COVID-19: A systematic review and meta-analysis. *Travel Medicine and Infectious Disease, 34*, 101623. Available from https://doi.org/10.1016/j.tmaid.2020.101623. Epub 2020 Mar 13.

Rosas, I. O., Bräu, N., Waters, M., Go, R. C., Hunter, B. D., Bhagani, S., Skiest, D., Aziz, M. S., Cooper, N., Douglas, I. S., Savic, S., Youngstein, T., Sorbo, L. D., Gracian, A. C., De La Zerda, D. J., Ustianowski, A., Bao, M., Dimonaco, S., Graham, E., ... Malhotra, A. (2021). Tocilizumab in hospitalized patients with severe Covid-19 pneumonia. *New England Journal of Medicine, 384*(16), 1503–1516. Available from https://doi.org/10.1056/nejmoa2028700.

Rothe, C., Schunk, M., Sothmann, P., Bretzel, G., Froeschl, G., Wallrauch, C., Zimmer, T., Thiel, V., Janke, C., Guggemos, W., Seilmaier, M., Drosten, C., Vollmar, P., Zwirglmaier, K., Zange, S., Wölfel, R., & Hoelscher, M. (2020). Transmission of 2019-NCOV infection from an asymptomatic contact in Germany. *New England Journal of Medicine, 382*(10), 970–971. Available from https://doi.org/10.1056/NEJMc2001468.

Ruscitti, P., Berardicurti, O., Iagnocco, A., & Giacomelli, R. (2020). Cytokine storm syndrome in severe COVID-19. *Autoimmunity Reviews, 19*(7), 102562.

Russmann, S., Grattagliano, I., Portincasa, P., Palmieri, V. O., & Palasciano, G. (2006). Ribavirin-induced anemia: Mechanisms, risk factors and related targets for future research. *Current Medicinal Chemistry, 13*(27), 3351–3357. Available from https://doi.org/10.2174/092986706778773059.

Sahlin, J. J., & Peppas, N. A. (1997). Enhanced hydrogel adhesion by polymer interdiffusion: Use of linear poly(ethylene glycol) as an adhesion promoter. *Journal of Biomaterials Science, Polymer Edition, 8*(6), 421–436. Available from https://doi.org/10.1163/156856297X00362.

Salama, C., Han, J., Yau, L., Reiss, W. G., Kramer, B., Neidhart, J. D., Criner, G. J., Kaplan-Lewis, E., Baden, R., Pandit, L., Cameron, M. L., Garcia-Diaz, J., Chávez, V., Mekebeb-Reuter, M., De Menezes, F. L., Shah, R., González-Lara, M. F., Assman, B., Freedman, J., & Mohan, S. V. (2021). Tocilizumab in patients hospitalized with Covid-19 pneumonia. *New England Journal of Medicine, 384*(1), 20–30. Available from https://doi.org/10.1056/NEJMoa2030340.

Samaridou, E., Heyes, J., & Lutwyche, P. (2020). Lipid nanoparticles for nucleic acid delivery: Current perspectives. *Advanced Drug Delivery Reviews, 154–155*, 37–63. Available from https://doi.org/10.1016/j.addr.2020.06.002.

Sheahan, T. P., Sims, A. C., Leist, S. R., Schäfer, A., Won, J., Brown, A. J., Montgomery, S. A., Hogg, A., Babusis, D., Clarke, M. O., Spahn, J. E., Bauer, L., Sellers, S., Porter, D., Feng, J. Y., Cihlar, T., Jordan, R., Denison, M. R., & Baric, R. S. (2020). Comparative therapeutic efficacy of remdesivir and combination lopinavir, ritonavir, and interferon beta against MERS-CoV. *Nature Communications, 11*(1). Available from https://doi.org/10.1038/s41467-019-13940-6.

Shi, R., Shan, C., Duan, X., Chen, Z., Liu, P., Song, J., Song, T., Bi, X., Han, C., Wu, L., Gao, G., Hu, X., Zhang, Y., Tong, Z., Huang, W., Liu, W. J., Wu, G., Zhang, B., Wang, L., & Yan, J. (2020). A human neutralizing antibody targets the receptor-binding site of SARS-CoV-2. *Nature, 584*(7819), 120–124. Available from https://doi.org/10.1038/s41586-020-2381-y.

Si, Y., Wen, Y., Kelly, S. H., Chong, A. S., & Collier, J. H. (2018). Intranasal delivery of adjuvant-free peptide nanofibers elicits resident CD8 + T cell responses. *Journal of Controlled Release, 282*, 120–130. Available from https://doi.org/10.1016/j.jconrel.2018.04.031.

Smith, T. R. F., Patel, A., Ramos, S., Elwood, D., Zhu, X., Yan, J., Gary, E. N., Walker, S. N., Schultheis, K., Purwar, M., Xu, Z., Walters, J., Bhojnagarwala, P., Yang, M., Chokkalingam, N., Pezzoli, P., Parzych, E., Reuschel, E. L., Doan, A., & Broderick, K. E. (2020). Immunogenicity of a DNA vaccine candidate for COVID-19. *Nature Communications, 11*(1). Available from https://doi.org/10.1038/s41467-020-16505-0.

Sogut, O., Can, M. M., Guven, R., Kaplan, O., Ergenc, H., Umit, T. B., Demir, O., Kaya, M., Akdemir, T., & Cakmak, S. (2021). Safety and efficacy of hydroxychloroquine in 152 outpatients with confirmed COVID-19: A pilot observational study. *American Journal of Emergency Medicine, 40*, 41–46. Available from https://doi.org/10.1016/j.ajem.2020.12.014.

Spruth, M., Kistner, O., Savidis-Dacho, H., Hitter, E., Crowe, B., Gerencer, M., Brühl, P., Grillberger, L., Reiter, M., Tauer, C., Mundt, W., & Barrett, P. N. (2006). A double-inactivated whole virus candidate SARS coronavirus vaccine stimulates neutralising and protective antibody responses. *Vaccine*, *24*(5), 652–661. Available from https://doi.org/10.1016/j.vaccine.2005.08.055.

Sun, X., Wang, T., Cai, D., Hu, Z., Chen, J., Liao, H., Zhi, L., Wei, H., Zhang, Z., Qiu, Y., Wang, J., & Wang, A. (2020). Cytokine storm intervention in the early stages of COVID-19 pneumonia. *Cytokine and Growth Factor Reviews*, *53*, 38–42. Available from https://doi.org/10.1016/j.cytogfr.2020.04.002.

Surya, W., Li, Y., Verdià-Bàguena, C., Aguilella, V. M., & Torres, J. (2015). MERS coronavirus envelope protein has a single transmembrane domain that forms pentameric ion channels. *Virus Research*, *201*, 61–66. Available from https://doi.org/10.1016/j.virusres.2015.02.023.

Tai, W., He, L., Zhang, X., Pu, J., Voronin, D., Jiang, S., Zhou, Y., & Du, L. (2020). Characterization of the receptor-binding domain (RBD) of 2019 novel coronavirus: implication for development of RBD protein as a viral attachment inhibitor and vaccine. *Cellular and Molecular Immunology*, *17*(6), 613–620. Available from https://doi.org/10.1038/s41423-020-0400-4.

Tallapaka, S. B., Karuturi, B. V. K., Yeapuri, P., Curran, S. M., Sonawane, Y. A., Phillips, J. A., David Smith, D., Sanderson, S. D., & Vetro, J. A. (2019). Surface conjugation of EP67 to biodegradable nanoparticles increases the generation of long-lived mucosal and systemic memory T-cells by encapsulated protein vaccine after respiratory immunization and subsequent T-cell-mediated protection against respiratory infection. *International Journal of Pharmaceutics*, *565*, 242–257. Available from https://doi.org/10.1016/j.ijpharm.2019.05.012.

Tian, Y., & Mao, S. (2012). Amphiphilic polymeric micelles as the nanocarrier for peroral delivery of poorly soluble anticancer drugs. *Expert Opinion on Drug Delivery*, *9*(6), 687–700. Available from https://doi.org/10.1517/17425247.2012.681299.

Tseng, C. T., Sbrana, E., Iwata-Yoshikawa, N., Newman, P. C., Garron, T., Atmar, R. L., Peters, C. J., & Couch, R. B. (2012). Immunization with SARS coronavirus vaccines leads to pulmonary immunopathology on challenge with the SARS virus. *PLoS ONE*, 7(4). Available from https://doi.org/10.1371/journal.pone.0035421.

Vetter, V., Denizer, G., Friedland, L. R., Krishnan, J., & Shapiro, M. (2018). Understanding modern-day vaccines: what you need to know. *Annals of Medicine*, *50* (2), 110–120. Available from https://doi.org/10.1080/07853890.2017.1407035.

Wagstaff, K. M., Sivakumaran, H., Heaton, S. M., Harrich, D., & Jans, D. A. (2012). Ivermectin is a specific inhibitor of importin α/β-mediated nuclear import able to inhibit replication of HIV-1 and dengue virus. *Biochemical Journal*, *443*(3), 851–856. Available from https://doi.org/10.1042/BJ20120150.

Walls, A. C., Fiala, B., Schäfer, A., Wrenn, S., Pham, M. N., Murphy, M., Tse, L. V, Shehata, L., O'Connor, M. A., Chen, C., Navarro, M. J., Miranda, M. C., Pettie, D., Ravichandran, R., Kraft, J. C., Ogohara, C., Palser, A., Chalk, S., Lee, E.-C., Kepl, E., Chow, C. M., Sydeman, C., Hodge, E. A., Brown, B., Fuller, J. T., Dinnon, K. H. 3rd, Gralinski, L. E., Leist, S. R., Gully, K. L., Lewis, T. B., Guttman, M., Chu, H. Y., Lee, K. K., Fuller, D. H., Baric, R. S., Kellam, P., Carter, L., Pepper, M., Sheahan, T. P., Veesler, D., King, N. P., 2020. Elicitation of potent neutralizing antibody responses by designed protein nanoparticle vaccines for SARS-CoV-2. Cell *183* (5), 1367–1382.e17 Available from https://doi.org/10.1101/2020.08.11.247395.

Walsh, E. E., Frenck, R. W., Falsey, A. R., Kitchin, N., Absalon, J., Gurtman, A., Lockhart, S., Neuzil, K., Mulligan, M. J., Bailey, R., Swanson, K. A., Li, P., Koury, K., Kalina, W., Cooper, D., Fontes-Garfias, C., Shi, P. Y., Türeci, Ö., Tompkins, K. R., & Gruber, W. C. (2020). Safety and immunogenicity of two RNA-based covid-19 vaccine candidates. *New England Journal of Medicine*, *383*(25), 2439–2450. Available from https://doi.org/10.1056/NEJMoa2027906.

Wang, D., Hu, B., Hu, C., Zhu, F., Liu, X., Zhang, J., Wang, B., Xiang, H., Cheng, Z., Xiong, Y., Zhao, Y., Li, Y., Wang, X., & Peng, Z. (2020). Clinical characteristics of 138 hospitalized patients with 2019 Novel Coronavirus-infected pneumonia in Wuhan, China. *JAMA – Journal of the American Medical Association*, *323*(11), 1061–1069. Available from https://doi.org/10.1001/jama.2020.1585.

Wang, J., Wang, Y., Wu, L., Wang, X., Jin, Z., Gao, Z., & Wang, Z. (2020). Ruxolitinib for refractory/relapsed hemophagocytic lymphohistiocytosis. *Haematologica*, *105*(5), E210–E212. Available from https://doi.org/10.3324/HAEMATOL.2019.222471.

Wang, M., Cao, R., Zhang, L., Yang, X., Liu, J., Xu, M., Shi, Z., Hu, Z., Zhong, W., & Xiao, G. (2020). Remdesivir and chloroquine effectively inhibit the recently emerged novel coronavirus (2019-nCoV) in vitro. *Cell Research*, *30*(3), 269–271. Available from https://doi.org/10.1038/s41422-020-0282-0.

Wang, N., Chen, M., & Wang, T. (2019). Liposomes used as a vaccine adjuvant-delivery system: From basics to clinical immunization. *Journal of Controlled Release*, *303*, 130–150. Available from https://doi.org/10.1016/j.jconrel.2019.04.025.

Weingartl, H., Czub, M., Czub, S., Neufeld, J., Marszal, P., Gren, J., Smith, G., Jones, S., Proulx, R., Deschambault, Y., Grudeski, E., Andonov, A., He, R., Li, Y., Copps, J., Grolla, A., Dick, D., Berry, J., Ganske, S., & Cao, J. (2004). Immunization with modified vaccinia virus Ankara-based recombinant vaccine against severe acute respiratory syndrome is associated with enhanced hepatitis in ferrets. *Journal of Virology*, *78*(22), 12672–12676. Available from https://doi.org/10.1128/JVI.78.22.12672-12676.2004.

Weinreich, D. M., Sivapalasingam, S., Norton, T., Ali, S., Gao, H., Bhore, R., Musser, B. J., Soo, Y., Rofail, D., Im, J., Perry, C., Pan, C., Hosain, R., Mahmood, A., Davis, J. D., Turner, K. C., Hooper, A. T., Hamilton, J. D., Baum, A., & Yancopoulos, G. D. (2021). REGN-COV2, a neutralizing antibody cocktail, in outpatients with Covid-19. *New England Journal of Medicine*, *384*(3), 238–251. Available from https://doi.org/10.1056/NEJMoa2035002.

Wilson, K. D., de Jong, S. D., & Tam, Y. K. (2009). Lipid-based delivery of CpG oligonucleotides enhances immunotherapeutic efficacy. *Advanced Drug Delivery Reviews*, *61* (3), 233–242. Available from https://doi.org/10.1016/j.addr.2008.12.014.

Woods, A. S., & Ferré, S. (2005). Amazing stability of the arginine-phosphate electrostatic interaction. *Journal of Proteome Research*, *4*(4), 1397–1402. Available from https://doi.org/10.1021/pr050077s.

World Health Organization. (2020). Laboratory testing for coronavirus disease (COVID-19) in suspected human cases: interim guidance, 19 March 2020. https://apps.who.int/iris/handle/10665/331501. License: CC BY-NC-SA 3.0 IGO.

Xiang, S. D., Wilson, K. L., Goubier, A., Heyerick, A., & Plebanski, M. (2018). Design of peptide-based nanovaccines targeting leading antigens from gynecological cancers to induce HLA-A2.1 restricted CD8+ T cell responses. *Frontiers in Immunology*, *9* (2968). Available from https://doi.org/10.3389/fimmu.2018.02968.

Xu, Z., Shi, L., Wang, Y., Zhang, J., Huang, L., Zhang, C., Liu, S., Zhao, P., Liu, H., Zhu, L., Tai, Y., Bai, C., Gao, T., Song, J., Xia, P., Dong, J., Zhao, J., & Wang, F. S. (2020). Pathological findings of COVID-19 associated with acute respiratory distress syndrome. *The Lancet Respiratory Medicine*, *8*(4), 420–422. Available from https://doi.org/10.1016/S2213-2600(20)30076-X.

Yan, W., Chen, W., & Huang, L. (2007). Mechanism of adjuvant activity of cationic liposome: Phosphorylation of a MAP kinase, ERK and induction of chemokines. *Molecular Immunology*, *44*(15), 3672–3681. Available from https://doi.org/10.1016/j.molimm.2007.04.009.

Yang, J., Bei, J., & Wang, S. (2002). Enhanced cell affinity of poly (D,L-lactide) by combining plasma treatment with collagen anchorage. *Biomaterials*, *23*(12), 2607–2614. Available from https://doi.org/10.1016/S0142-9612(01)00400-8.

Yang, L., Li, W., Kirberger, M., Liao, W., & Ren, J. (2016). Design of nanomaterial based systems for novel vaccine development. *Biomaterials Science, 4*(5), 785–802. Available from https://doi.org/10.1039/c5bm00507h.

Yang, Y., Ding, Y., Fan, B., Wang, Y., Mao, Z., Wang, W., & Wu, J. (2020). Inflammation-targeting polymeric nanoparticles deliver sparfloxacin and tacrolimus for combating acute lung sepsis. *Journal of Controlled Release, 321*, 463–474. Available from https://doi.org/10.1016/j.jconrel.2020.02.030.

Yue, Z. G., Wei, W., Lv, P. P., Yue, H., Wang, L. Y., Su, Z. G., & Ma, G. H. (2011). Surface charge affects cellular uptake and intracellular trafficking of chitosan-based nanoparticles. *Biomacromolecules, 12*(7), 2440–2446. Available from https://doi.org/10.1021/bm101482r.

Yusuf, H., Ali, A. A., Orr, N., Tunney, M. M., McCarthy, H. O., & Kett, V. L. (2017). Novel freeze-dried DDA and TPGS liposomes are suitable for nasal delivery of vaccine. *International Journal of Pharmaceutics, 533*(1), 179–186. Available from https://doi.org/10.1016/j.ijpharm.2017.09.011.

Zhang, C., Wu, Z., Li, J. W., Zhao, H., & Wang, G. Q. (2020). Cytokine release syndrome in severe COVID-19: interleukin-6 receptor antagonist tocilizumab may be the key to reduce mortality. *International Journal of Antimicrobial Agents, 55*(5), 105954.

Zhang, S., Huang, S., Lu, L., Song, X., Li, P., & Wang, F. (2018). Curdlan sulfate-O-linked quaternized chitosan nanoparticles: Potential adjuvants to improve the immunogenicity of exogenous antigens via intranasal vaccination. *International Journal of Nanomedicine, 13*, 2377–2394. Available from https://doi.org/10.2147/IJN.S158536.

Zhang, S., Jiang, H., Huang, S., Li, P., & Wang, F. (2019). Curdlan sulfate/O-linked quaternized chitosan nanoparticles acting as potential adjuvants promote multiple arms of immune responses. *Carbohydrate Polymers, 213*, 100–111. Available from https://doi.org/10.1016/j.carbpol.2019.02.093.

Zhou, P., Yang, X. L., Wang, X. G., Hu, B., Zhang, L., Zhang, W., Si, H. R., Zhu, Y., Li, B., Huang, C. L., Chen, H. D., Chen, J., Luo, Y., Guo, H., Jiang, R. D., Liu, M. Q., Chen, Y., Shen, X. R., Wang, X., & Shi, Z. L. (2020). A pneumonia outbreak associated with a new coronavirus of probable bat origin. *Nature, 579*(7798), 270–273. Available from https://doi.org/10.1038/s41586-020-2012-7.

Zhu, F. C., Li, Y. H., Guan, X. H., Hou, L. H., Wang, W. J., Li, J. X., Wu, S. P., Wang, B. S., Wang, Z., Wang, L., Jia, S. Y., Jiang, H. D., Wang, L., Jiang, T., Hu, Y., Gou, J. B., Xu, S. B., Xu, J. J., Wang, X. W., & Chen, W. (2020). Safety, tolerability, and immunogenicity of a recombinant adenovirus type-5 vectored COVID-19 vaccine: a dose-escalation, open-label, non-randomised, first-in-human trial. *The Lancet, 395*(10240), 1845–1854. Available from https://doi.org/10.1016/S0140-6736(20)31208-3.

Zhu, Z., Lu, Z., Xu, T., Chen, C., Yang, G., Zha, T., Lu, J., & Xue, Y. (2020). Arbidol monotherapy is superior to lopinavir/ritonavir in treating COVID-19. *Journal of Infection, 81*(1), e21–e23. Available from https://doi.org/10.1016/j.jinf.2020.03.060.

Zhuang, Y., Ma, Y., Wang, C., Hai, L., Yan, C., Zhang, Y., Liu, F., & Cai, L. (2012). PEGylated cationic liposomes robustly augment vaccine-induced immune responses: Role of lymphatic trafficking and biodistribution. *Journal of Controlled Release, 159*(1), 135–142. Available from https://doi.org/10.1016/j.jconrel.2011.12.017.

CHAPTER 3

Nanomaterials and immune system*

Nourhan Mohamed[1], Mahmoud Elsabahy[2,3,4], Karen L. Wooley[3] and Noura G. Eissa[5]
[1]Department of Microbiology and Immunology, Faculty of Pharmacy, Sphinx University, Assiut, Egypt
[2]School of Biotechnology and Science Academy, Badr University in Cairo, Badr City, Cairo, Egypt
[3]Department of Chemistry, Laboratory for Synthetic-Biologic Interactions, Texas A&M University, College Station, TX, United States
[4]Misr University for Science and Technology, 6th of October City, Giza, Egypt
[5]Department of Pharmaceutics and Industrial Pharmacy, Faculty of Pharmacy, Zagazig University, Zagazig, Egypt

3.1 Introduction

Nanomedicines are emerging as potential therapeutics and diagnostics for a wide variety of diseases and have also found uses in vaccine development, engineering, and materials science applications (Elsabahy & Wooley, 2012a,b; Nyström & Wooley, 2011; Von Maltzahn et al., 2011; Yoo et al., 2011). As a "depot" for various cargoes, they have been successfully used for the delivery of hydrophobic and hydrophilic small molecule drugs (e.g., anticancer drugs) and biomacromolecules, such as recombinant proteins, enzymes, hormones, peptides, and monoclonal antibodies. In addition, they have been used to deliver nucleic acids of various sizes and structures (Davis et al., 2010; Tacken et al., 2011; Zhang et al., 2009, 2010). The macro- and ultra-structures of these nanosized materials can be tailored to accommodate particular therapeutics and to protect them against hydrolytic or enzymatic degradation and provide the appropriate environment for solubility and for gated drug release. In addition, they can be equipped with "smart" components (antibodies, peptides, proteins, sugars, aptamers, etc.) to aid in their delivery to target organs, tissues, and subcellular compartments (Elsabahy & Wooley, 2012a,b; Nyström & Wooley, 2011; Von Maltzahn et al., 2011; Yoo et al., 2011). Several nanomedicine products are already on the market and in different

* Adapted from "Elsabahy, M., & Wooley, K. L. (2013). Cytokines as biomarkers of nanoparticle immunotoxicity. *Chemical Society Reviews, 42*(12), 5552–5576. https://doi.org/10.1039/C3CS60064E.

Immunomodulatory Effects of Nanomaterials
DOI: https://doi.org/10.1016/B978-0-323-90604-3.00005-X

phases of clinical trials, and many more are still under rigorous investigation, optimization, and screening to select the most promising candidates for therapeutic and diagnostic applications.

Nanoparticles can interact with various components of the immune system and either enhance or inhibit its function (Dobrovolskaia & McNeil, 2007; Dobrovolskaia et al., 2009; Hussain et al., 2012; Zolnik et al., 2010). Modulation of the immune function by nanomaterials can be useful or detrimental, depending on the intended use (Zolnik et al., 2010). Nanoparticles can be designed to be immunomodulatory to serve specific functions (e.g., vaccine adjuvants, antiinflammatory, immunosuppressive drugs). Concerns are raised, however, when an engineered nanomaterial not intended for interaction with the immune system alters its function. It has been established that certain nanomaterials can be immunotoxic, although no standard immunotoxicity assay has been described thus far that is specific to their nano size (Chang, 2010; Dobrovolskaia & McNeil, 2007; Dwivedi et al., 2011; Hussain et al., 2012; Zolnik et al., 2010). It is generally agreed that the same set of immunological studies routinely used to assess immunotoxicity of chemicals, medical devices, and drugs can be applied to engineered nanomaterials (Dobrovolskaia et al., 2009).

Cytokines are proteins produced by various types of cells including immune cells in response to activation. They play a pivotal role in homeostasis by both modulating and regulating the immune response. Cytokine functions are pleiotropic, in that they perform multiple actions and often overlap, acting synergistically or antagonizing each other. This is why cytokine interactions are often referred to as a network. Cytokine release can be characterized by fever, hypotension, nausea, headache, chills, vomiting, and muscle pain and is the cause of infusion reactions commonly associated with antibody-based biotherapeutics (Breslin, 2007), which, in some cases, may be life-threatening (Schneider et al., 2006). Hence, it became a common practice in the pharmaceutical industry to monitor cytokines in preclinical studies to understand, prevent, and control undesirable cytokine responses to biotherapeutics.

As nanoparticles can interact with proteins, and proteins, including antibodies, are often used to target nanoparticles to specific cells and tissues, understanding the use of cytokines as biomarkers of undesirable immunostimulation associated with engineered nanomaterials is emerging as an essential component of nanoparticle safety testing. Evaluation of the immunotoxicity of nanomaterials by measuring the levels of cytokines, in particular the proinflammatory cytokines, can be useful tools in evaluating nanoparticle immunotoxicity. High levels of cytokines upon treatment with nanoparticles are usually associated with toxicity, adverse reactions, and low therapeutic efficacy, as will be discussed later. Hence, cytokines might be utilized to partially predict nanoparticle immunotoxicity.

Here, we review the possible interactions between the various components of nanomaterials and the immune system with respect to the induction of cytokines. We highlight studies demonstrating the utility of cytokines as biomarkers of both desirable immunostimulation and undesirable immunotoxicity of engineered nanomaterials. In addition, the rational design of nanomaterials with low immunogenicity and high therapeutic efficacy is discussed, with special attention to chemical modifications to both drugs and the nanoparticle-forming constituents utilized for their delivery.

3.2 The immune system

3.2.1 Structure of the immune system

The immune system has a complex architecture comprised of various organs and cell types that interact and communicate via chemical conductors to orchestrate an immune response toward a particular event (Box 3.1 and Fig. 3.1). The parts of the immune system are connected via the blood and lymphatic circulatory systems. Bone marrow, thymus, spleen, lymph nodes, and mucosa-associated lymphoid tissues are the main organs of the immune system, which are involved in the manufacturing, maturation, differentiation, proliferation, and storage of immune cells. The blood is composed of red blood cells and white blood cells, which are suspended in the blood together with other molecules, such as various complement proteins and immunoglobulins. White blood cells (leukocytes), which play a major role in the immune system, are mainly made up of polymorphonuclear granulocytes (PMNs), in addition to monocytes, natural killer (NK) cells, and B and T lymphocytes. PMNs are composed mainly of neutrophils (phagocytic cells), along with eosinophils and basophils. T and B lymphocytes, natural killer cells, and PMNs are the main cells of the immune system. In addition, dendritic cells and macrophages are essential parts of the immune system that act as scavengers or antigen-presenting cells (APCs). Mononuclear phagocytic system (MPS) is the name given to the part of the immune system that consists of phagocytic cells, such as blood monocytes and macrophages accumulated in lymph nodes, liver, spleen, and other tissues (Box 3.1).

Innate and adaptive immunity refer to inborn and acquired immune defense lines, respectively. Innate immunity is rapid and provides a first-line

BOX 3.1 The immune system

Organs of the immune system: *Bone marrow, thymus, spleen, lymph nodes, and mucosa-associated lymphoid tissues*. During hematopoiesis, bone marrow-derived stem cells differentiate into either mature cells or into precursors of cells that migrate out of the bone marrow to continue their maturation elsewhere, for example, maturation of T lymphocytes occurs in the thymus. The spleen acts as an immunologic filter of the blood, whereas the nodes filter the tissue fluids (i.e., lymph). The mucosa-associated lymphoid tissues are aggregates of lymphoid tissues near the mucosal surfaces.

Cells of the immune system: Leukocytes (white blood cells) consist of the following: (1) polymorphonuclear granulocytes (PMN): neutrophils, eosinophils, and basophils; (2) monocytes: can be differentiated into macrophages; (3) natural killer cells; (4) B lymphocytes: produce antibodies; and (5) T lymphocytes: T helper cells, suppressor T cells, and cytotoxic T cells. Lymphocytes and mononuclear phagocytes play a central role in the immune response (Lanier, 1991).

Immune response: Antigen-presenting cells (APCs) are cells that are capable of processing an antigen and presenting part of it onto the MHC II where it can interact with the appropriate immune cell receptors. Dendritic cells, macrophages, and B cells are the main APCs for T cells, whereas follicular dendritic cells are the main APCs for B cells. APCs and B or T cells communicate together, either directly or via cytokines, to initiate an immune response. Antigen processing and presentation signal these cells to proliferate and secrete antibodies (B cells), cytokines ($CD4^+$), or become activated to kill cells expressing the antigen presented by the APC ($CD8^+$). The antibodies secreted by B cells can directly bind to that antigen, which accelerates the clearance by the PMNs or macrophages. The antibodies may also initiate the complement destruction cascade by attracting the serum protein to bind to the immobilized antibodies that are bound to the antigen, thereby aiding in the phagocytosis process and elimination of the immune complex.

Mononuclear phagocytic system (MPS): The original term used to refer to the phagocytic system is reticulo-endothelial system (RES). It refers to the mononuclear cells of mesenchymal origin that reside in the reticular organs including the liver, spleen, and lymph nodes and other organs and possess the collective property of rapidly engulfing colloids and particulate materials. As not all endothelial and reticular cells are phagocytic, the term RES was recently replaced with MPS; however, in the literature, RES and MPS are often used interchangeably. MPS is distributed throughout the body and is mainly responsible for the phagocytosis, clearance, and initiation of the immune response due to the introduction of the nanomaterials, foreign particles, or antigens in the body, and it also engulfs and clears aged cells in the blood

(*Continued*)

BOX 3.1 (Continued)

and tissues. Phagocytic cells include PMN, blood monocytes, and tissue macrophages (Kupffer cells in the liver, alveolar macrophages in the lung, splenic macrophages, peritoneal cells in the peritoneal fluids, microglial cells in the central nervous tissues, histiocytes of the connective tissues, and dendritic cells). These cells have a number of surface receptors that allow them to bind carbohydrates, complement proteins, and immunoglobulins. If the MHC II is expressed on the surface of the phagocytes, it enables them to function as APCs. Opsonins ("prepare food for") are antibodies, complement proteins, and other serum components that upon binding to foreign particles make them easier targets for phagocytes.

Complement system: It is a part of the immune system that comprises a biochemical proteolytic cascade that aids (complement) the antibodies and phagocytic cells to eliminate pathogens from the body.

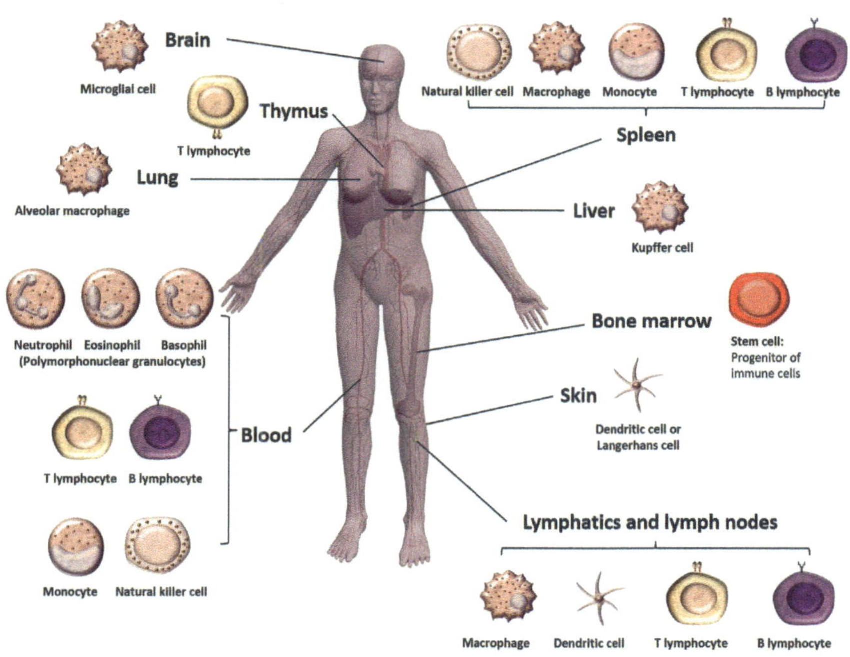

Figure 3.1 Human body showing the various organs of the immune system. Distribution of the various immune cells into the immune organs and other organs that are rich in macrophages.

defense, while an adaptive response is more involved and takes more time. Phagocytic cells, NK cells, and secondary messenger molecules (e.g., cytokines, eicosanoids, prostaglandins) produced in response to a pathogen challenge, as well as the complement system, are the major players in an innate immune response. The two main types of adaptive immune responses are cell-mediated and humoral- or antibody-mediated immunity, and they are mediated mainly by T and B lymphocytes. The interaction between innate and adaptive immunity is regulated through mediator molecules such as complement proteins and cytokines.

Phagocytic cells (e.g., monocytes, neutrophils, dendritic cells, B cells, platelets, and macrophages) can be found in the blood, skin, mucous membranes, and various organs, such as the liver, spleen, lymph nodes, lung, and brain (Box 3.1). Some of them (e.g., monocytes and neutrophils) roam through the body and act as scavengers to attack and engulf foreign particles, remove pathogens, old or dead cells, and synthesize complement proteins and cytokines that are essential for the synchronization of the various parts of the immune system. These cells may attack and engulf particles that are tagged by opsonins (adsorbed molecules that enhance or accelerate clearance by the immune system) or nonopsonized particles.

APCs engulf and digest foreign antigens and present fragments of the antigens on their surface-bound receptors, major histocompatibility complexes (MHCs), to other cells of the immune system such as T cells and B cells. There are two types of MHCs: MHC I, which are found in most of the body tissues, and MHC II, which are only present in the APCs. The MHC II receptors wrap the antigen and present it to T cell receptors (TCR), resulting in the activation of T cells. T lymphocytes confer cell-mediated immunity and cooperate with B cells, enabling them to secrete antibodies for specific antigens. T lymphocytes include T helper (T_H) cells, suppressor T cells, and cytotoxic T cells, with the categorization depending on the expressed surface protein. T_H cells express CD3 and CD4, whereas the suppressor and cytotoxic T cells express CD3 and CD8 receptors. The T cells also express other receptors, for example, TCR, which can identify a broad range of specific antigens presented on MHC molecules. The $CD4^+$ cells recognize antigens presented on the MHC II by the APCs, whereas $CD8^+$ cells recognize antigens on the MHC I. $CD4^+$ cells are T_H0 cells that differentiate into either T_H1 or T_H2 cells. T_H1 cells participate in cell-mediated immunity and regulate the steps of inflammation "T inflammatory cells," while T_H2 cells induce proliferation of mast cells and eosinophils and favor the differentiation of B cells to produce IgG and IgE, thereby promoting humoral immunity (Black, 1999; Rajananthanan et al., 1999). T_H1 cells secrete large quantities of interferon (IFN)-γ, interleukin (IL)-2, IL-3, granulocyte macrophage colony-stimulating factor (GM-CSF), and small quantities of tumor necrosis factor (TNF). T_H2 cells secrete large quantities of IL-3, IL-4, IL-5, IL-6, and IL-10 and small quantities of GM-CSF and TNF. The cytokines produced by specific T_H cells (e.g., IFN-γ from T_H1 cells and IL-10 from T_H2 cells) usually inhibit the action of another type of T cells and thereby potentiate a particular pattern of the immune response. IFN-γ and IL-4 are the main markers of T_H1 and T_H2 cells, respectively. It is accepted that the main function of T_H1 cells is to fight viruses and intracellular pathogens, while that of T_H2 cells is to control humoral response and extracellular pathogens. More recently, other subsets of T cells were discovered, which are distinct from T_H1 and T_H2 cells. They are T_H9 cells, which produce IL-9 and are involved in fighting parasites, T_H17 cells, which produce IL-17 and are involved in autoimmune response, and regulatory T cells (Tregs), characterized by the presence of FoxP3 and antigen-experienced follicular helper T cells, identified by expression of CXCR5 (Ma et al., 2010; Medzhitov et al., 2011). The TCR and B cell-bound antibodies recognize antigens and initiate an immune response by recruiting other immune cells, cytokines, and complement proteins.

3.2.2 Proinflammatory cytokines

The T_H1/T_H2 hypothesis, proposed more than 20 years ago, suggested that naïve $CD4^+$ T cells can differentiate into distinct subsets performing various functions to protect the host from certain pathogens (Mosmann et al., 1986). The initial studies that provided the background for the T_H1/T_H2 hypothesis were performed in mice and were later adopted in human cells. The balance between the T_H1 and T_H2 cytokines was thought to be clinically significant. Some studies have suggested that it should be evaluated (Wang et al., 2011), because this balance is also of particular importance to prevent the occurrence of several diseases (e.g., arthritis, diabetes, asthma, cancer) (Kidd, 2003; Kokkonen et al., 2010; Lan et al., 2011; Neurath et al., 2002; Nguyen & Casale, 2011; Wang et al., 2011). However, not all immune responses can be described through T_H1/T_H2 theory. For example, some substances (e.g., omega-3 fatty acids) have considerable effects on inflammatory and autoimmune conditions without a significant shift in T_H1/T_H2 balance, while other substances (e.g., melanin, probiotics, and zinc) affect T_H1/T_H2 balance but do not cause inflammatory and autoimmune diseases (Kidd, 2003). The limitations of this theory were further clarified by the discovery of other types of T effector cells (T_H9, T_H17, Tregs). However, despite this, the type of immunostimulation and its outcome to the host is still often judged by the T_H1 and T_H2 type cytokines, and most commercially available assays are aimed at the T_H1/T_H2 panel.

Many cytokines including IL-1, IL-6, and TNF-α activate the functions of inflammatory cells during acute inflammatory responses. These cytokines increase vascular permeability and thus cause swelling and redness associated with inflammation. IL-1 and IL-6 are responsible for fever reactions, TNF-α stimulates endothelial cells and is responsible for hypotension, IL-8 is a chemokine that plays a key role in the activation of neutrophils and their recruitment to the site of inflammation. Many cytokines act together to initiate and regulate the inflammation process. For example, IFN-γ plays a significant role in the inflammatory process, as it can attract macrophages to sites where antigens are present (Benjamini et al., 2000). Although T_H cells are the major source of cytokines that regulate the immune response, other cells, such as keratinocytes, can produce cytokines that serve as mediators of inflammatory and immunologic reactions in skin exposed to irritants (Davis et al., 2010; Tacken et al., 2011; Zhang et al., 2009, 2010). These cytokines can also affect the proliferation and differentiation of keratinocytes and control the production of other cytokines (Gröne, 2002). These proinflammatory cytokines have been well studied and characterized as participants in the basic inflammatory process and mediators of cellular infiltration (Beyerle et al., 2010; Cubillos-Ruiz et al., 2009; Kim et al., 2003; Powers et al., 2005; Ryman-Rasmussen et al., 2007; Zhang et al., 2008).

3.3 Nanomaterials

The structure and composition of nanoparticles can be tailored to carry drugs of various sizes and solubilities (Box 3.2 and Fig. 3.2) (Elsabahy & Wooley, 2012a,b). Nanoparticles can also be engineered to carry charged macromolecules (e.g., amino acids, nucleic acids, or enzymes). Attachment or encapsulation of these drugs into nanoparticles can improve their stability, protect them from systemic exposure and recognition by the immune system, and control their release. For certain types of

BOX 3.2 Nanomaterials in biomedicine

Nanomedicine: "The design of diagnostics and/or therapeutics on the nanoscale, which provides opportunities of coincident transport and delivery of the active species with mediation of their navigation within the biological systems for the treatment, prevention and diagnosis of diseases" (Elsabahy & Wooley, 2012a,b).

Types:

1. **Organic nanoparticles**:
   a. **Macromolecular conjugates (e.g., Xyotax, Oncaspar)**: Conjugating drug to a polymeric or lipidic segment to impart specific properties to the drug to facilitate or direct its delivery (Singer et al., 2005; Singer, 2005).
   b. **Nanoemulsions (e.g., Diprivan)**: Heterogeneous mixture of two immiscible liquids with an emulsifier that stabilizes the dispersed droplets. They can be utilized as carriers for hydrophilic or hydrophobic drugs for various therapeutic applications (Gianella et al., 2011; Stanberry et al., 2012).
   c. **Polymeric micelles (e.g., NK012, NK105, SP1049C, NC-6004, Genexol)**: Self-assembly of amphiphilic copolymer chains in an aqueous milieu presenting a core/shell architecture with a hydrophobic core and hydrophilic corona. Depending on the structure of the core-forming polymer and the forces driving the assembly, they may be classified also as polyion complex micelles or polymer–metal complex micelles (Gaucher et al., 2005; Kataoka et al., 2001; Torchilin, 2007).
   d. **Shell crosslinked knedel-like nanoparticles**: Shell crosslinked polymeric nanoparticles to enhance the kinetic stability and prevent the dissociation upon in vivo administration. Degradation of the core is also possible to form nanocages (Elsabahy & Wooley, 2012a; Nyström & Wooley, 2011; Von Maltzahn et al., 2011; Yoo et al., 2011).
   e. **Protein-based and polymeric nanoparticles (e.g., Abraxane, BIND-014)**: Colloidal particles with a rigid core that are either made from a polymeric or lipidic matrix in which a drug is dissolved or dispersed or from drug nanocrystals stabilized by a polymer (Fuhrmann et al., 2012; Hawkins et al., 2008; Shi et al., 2011). Polymer brushes, unimolecular (e.g., dendrimers), and hyperbranched structures utilized for drug delivery may also fall into this category (Li & Wallace, 2008; Wolfrum et al., 2007).
   f. **Liposomes (e.g., Doxil, DaunoXome, Ambisome)**: Spherical vesicles composed of lipid bilayers and a hydrophilic core with the capability of solubilizing both hydrophilic and lipophilic drugs into the core and

(*Continued*)

BOX 3.2 (Continued)

lipid bilayers, respectively (Bedi et al., 2011; Movassaghian et al., 2011; Simard & Leroux, 2010).

g. **Lipoplexes and polyplexes (e.g., ALN-VSP)**: Complexes between nucleic acids (DNA/RNA) and cationic lipids or polymers, and when PEGylated are categorized as PEGylated lipoplexes and polyion complex micelles, respectively (Elsabahy et al., 2009; 2011; Nishiyama & Kataoka, 2006; Wolff & Rozema, 2008). Stable nucleic acid lipid particles may also fall into this category (Judge et al., 2009; Semple et al., 2010).

2. **Inorganic nanoparticles**:
   a. **Metal and metal-oxide nanoparticles**:
      i. **Gold nanoparticles (e.g., Aurimune)**: Nanoparticles that display interesting optical and electrical properties (Dreaden et al., 2011).
      ii. **Magnetic nanoparticles (Ferridex, Ferumoxytol, Resovist)**: Nanoparticles with magnetic properties (e.g., paramagnetic iron oxide nanoparticles) (Huang et al., 2011; Lee et al., 2009).
      iii. **Other nanoparticles**: Other kinds of nanoparticles do also exist, such as titanium oxide and platinum- and diamond-based nanoparticles.
   b. **Carbon nanotubes**: single-wall or multiwall cylindrical graphene sheets (Huang et al., 2011; Liu et al., 2008; Prato et al., 2008).
   c. **Quantum dots**: Inorganic semiconductor nanoparticles that are widely used as fluorophores for biological imaging (Huang et al., 2011).

engineered nanomaterials, coating with hydrophilic polymers may impart further protection against the external environment and increase blood circulation times. The coating is a nonionic hydrophilic flexible shell that prevents the adsorption of opsonins, thereby limiting uptake by the MPS and prolonging the circulation half-life of the encapsulated drug. Prolonged circulation times allow for passive targeting of the nanoparticles into tumors via the enhanced permeation and retention (EPR) effect (Fig. 3.3). The EPR effect is explained by the leaky vasculature and impaired lymphatic drainage at tumor sites, which results in the deposition of colloidal particles in tumor peripheries. Once deposited in tissues, the hydrophilic corona facilitates the transport of the nanomedicine through the extracellular matrix. Nanoparticles have also been decorated with targeting ligands to allow specific cellular uptake or direct the delivery system to a diseased site, and to circumvent various physiological barriers

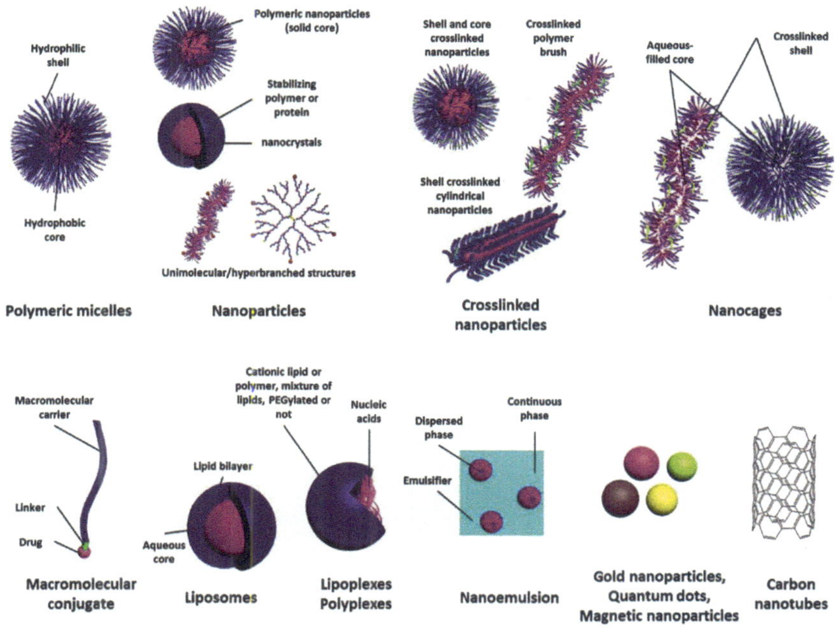

Figure 3.2 Common nanoparticulates utilized for delivery of a wide range of therapeutics. Brief explanation of each category is indicated in Box 4.2.

(Fig. 3.3) (Von Maltzahn et al., 2011). They can also be equipped with pH- or thermo-responsive (i.e., smart) components to allow the release of the drug only in diseased tissues, thereby reducing the toxicity to healthy tissues (Elsabahy & Wooley, 2012a,b; Felber et al., 2012).

Nanoparticles of different structures and compositions have been developed for biomedical delivery applications, such as polymeric, lipidic, metallic, and graphite-based nanoparticles (Box 3.2 and Fig. 3.2) (Kim et al., 2003; Ryman-Rasmussen et al., 2007; Zhang et al., 2008). Much focus has been given to the design of nanoparticles with tailored properties that can accommodate drugs of various sizes, structures, and physicochemical properties and to allow them to circulate for long times in the blood and to circumvent the various physiological barriers encountered on the way to the target sites, and to overcome cellular and subcellular barriers (Elsabahy & Wooley, 2012a). In addition, careful design of the various components of these nanosized particles to reduce toxicity and to enhance biocompatibility of nanoparticles has been shown to significantly enhance the safety of these formulations. For instance, the use of neutral hydrophilic layers on the surface of various nanostructures (e.g., nanocrystals,

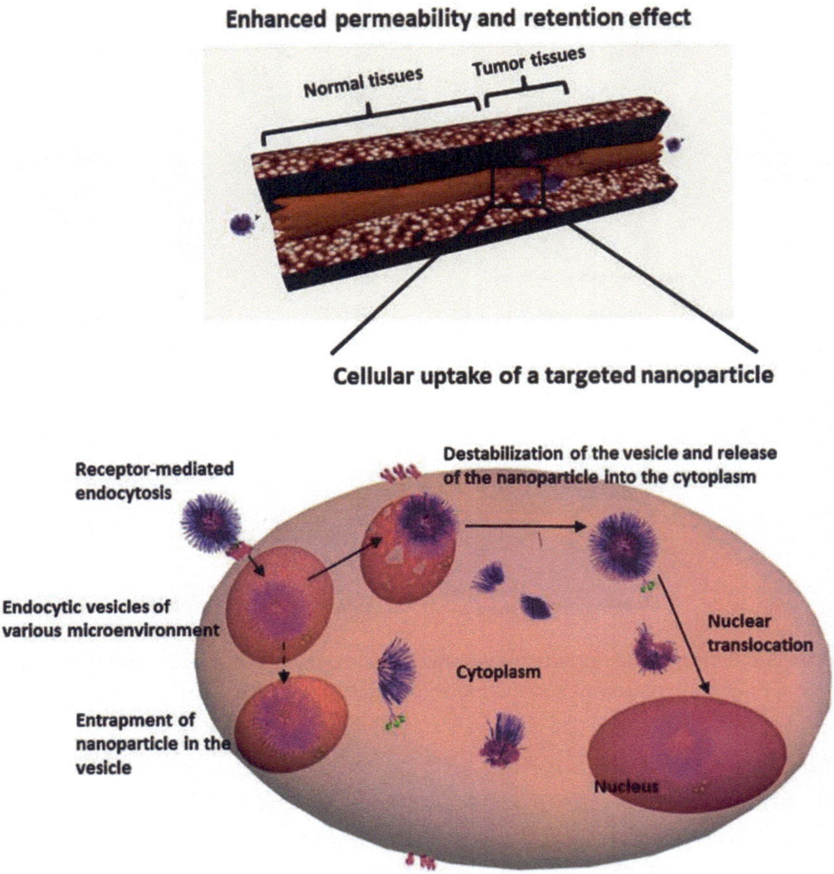

Figure 3.3 Passive and active targeting features of multifunctional nanomaterials. In passive targeting, nanoparticles accumulate into pathological sites with leaky vasculature (e.g., tumor) due to the enhanced permeability and retention effect. In active targeting, the targeting ligands on the surface of nanoparticles enhance cellular uptake by binding to specific receptors overexpressed on the diseased cells and can also be achieved via facilitating the escape from endosomes and/or enhancing nuclear translocation. Multifunctional nanoparticles have additional functionalities to deliver more than one cargo (e.g., more than one type of therapeutic and/or diagnostic), or combine more than one targeting mechanism (i.e., passive and active targeting). *From Elsabahy, M., & Wooley, K. L. (2012). Design of polymeric nanoparticles for biomedical delivery applications.* Chemical Society Reviews, 41, *2545–2561. Reproduced by permission of the Royal Society of Chemistry.*

polymeric, or lipidic drug complexes) has been shown to reduce the toxicity of these formulations by limiting the interactions of core components and biomacromolecules.

The benefits of using nanotechnology platforms for drug delivery are often challenged by concerns regarding the safety of these materials. Nanoparticle interactions with components of the immune system represent one category of safety concerns. The potential immunomodulatory effects of nanoparticles need to be understood to estimate whether or not nanomaterials are capable of inducing adverse reactions and complications. Information regarding nanoparticle immunotoxicity is also needed to ensure that interactions with the immune system will not affect the therapeutic efficacy of these nanotherapeutics (Hyde et al., 2008; Tan et al., 1999). Interactions between the various types of nanoparticles (organic and inorganic) and various components of the immune system, including plasma proteins have been described elsewhere (Chang, 2010; Dobrovolskaia & McNeil, 2007; Dobrovolskaia et al., 2009; Dwivedi et al., 2011; Hussain et al., 2012; Zolnik et al., 2010). However, at the time when these reports were prepared, the role of cytokines in nanoparticle-mediated immune responses had not been investigated in depth. This chapter presents a comprehensive overview of the currently available literature on this subject, with a focus on engineered nanomaterials.

3.4 Cytokines as biomarkers of immunomodulatory properties of nanomaterials

The ability of nanoparticles to induce an immune response (immunogenicity) is a product of the nanoparticles' physicochemical properties (size, charge, hydrophobicity, etc.). It is also influenced by other factors such as the surface targeting moieties and therapeutic payload, the animal model, and the route of administration. Nanoparticles can reach systemic circulation via different sites, where the route of administration plays a pivotal role in dictating the fate of the nanomaterials and their immunotoxicity (Fig. 3.4). The immune system may recognize many of the components of nanoparticles (e.g., shell, core, surface-decorating moieties, and cargoes) as foreign and initiates an immune response through a complex process.

There are several markers and measures, which can be utilized to study and predict the immune response of biomaterials, such as lymphocyte proliferation, cell surface markers, morphological and histopathological examination. Soluble mediators, such as antibodies (e.g., IgG, IgE, IgM), complement proteins (e.g., C3a, C5a), and cytokines (e.g., T_H1 and T_H2 cytokines) have also been exploited to evaluate the immunogenicity of various therapeutics. This review focuses on utilizing cytokines as biomarkers for

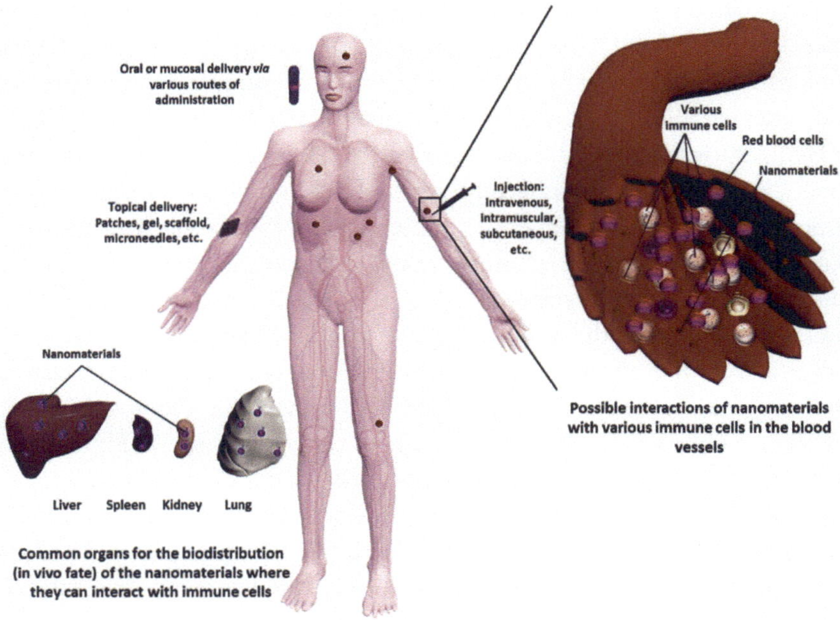

Figure 3.4 The possible interactions of nanoparticles with immune system. Nanoparticles interactions with the various components of the immune system after entering the body via various routes of administration (oral, mucosal, systemic, or topical).

nanoparticles immunotoxicity. However, the selection of the functional assay and biomarkers depends on several factors, such as the structure and composition of the medical device, route of administration, and therapeutic application. Combination of several markers might also be useful to understand the underlying mechanisms of immunotoxicity induced by nanomaterials.

3.4.1 Proinflammatory cytokines as biomarkers of nanoparticle immunotoxicity

The proinflammatory cytokines are often measured to predict the immunomodulatory effects of nanomaterials and the possibility of inflammation-mediated toxicity. They may also alter the therapeutic outcomes of the active pharmaceutical ingredients delivered through nanomaterials. The administration of nanoparticles may polarize the balance between the T_H1 and T_H2 cytokines toward one specific pathway (Huang et al., 2011; Liu et al., 2008; Prato et al., 2008). For instance, administration of polyhydroxylated metallofullerenol polarized the cytokine balance toward T_H1

cytokines via decreasing the production of T_H2 cytokines (IL-4, IL-5, and IL-6), and increasing the production of T_H1 cytokines (IL- 2, IFN-γ and TNF-α) in the serum of the treated mice (Liu et al., 2009). In another study, systemic administration of cationic protamine DNA lipoplexes to mice resulted in the production of large amounts of proinflammatory cytokines (TNF-α, IL1-β, IL-12, and IFN-γ) (Tan et al., 1999). These cytokines were associated both with toxicities in animals and inhibition of transgene expression (short duration of gene expression and refractoriness to repeated dosing at frequent intervals). The inhibition of gene expression was tested by preinjection of the vehicle and was correlated with the levels of cytokines production. In addition, intraperitoneal injection of dexamethasone suppressed cytokine production and led to higher levels of transgene expression. As commonly recognized, the unmethylated cytosine—phosphate—guanine (CpG) motifs, especially when combined with cationic vehicles, are responsible for immunomodulatory effects. It was reported that polyethyleneimine (PEI) (linear in vivo-jetPEI), a commonly utilized cationic polymer for nucleic acid delivery, is a selective TLR5 agonist and can elicit the production of TLR5-inducible cytokines in a dose-dependent manner, whereas no secretion of these cytokines was found in the *Tlr5*$^{-/-}$ mice (Cubillos-Ruiz et al., 2009). Intraperitoneal administration of PEI to mice induced significant and selective upregulation of the chemokine KC (the mouse functional homolog of human IL-8) (Kim et al., 2003; Powers et al., 2005) 2-h after injection (Cubillos-Ruiz et al., 2009). In another study, increased levels of IL-6 and G-CSF were detected after treatment with PEGylated PEI (branched PEI, molecular weight = 25 kDa) (Powers et al., 2005). However, further studies are still required to understand the detailed mechanisms of these immunomodulatory patterns and the particular specificity to PEI. The release of proinflammatory cytokines has also been observed with inorganic nanoparticles of various types and morphologies (titanium dioxide (TiO_2), nanodiamond, and nanoplatinum) in addition to other manifestations of immunotoxicity, such as dendritic cell maturation and activation and proliferation of naïve T cells (Ghoneum et al., 2010; Schanen et al., 2009).

Nanoparticle-induced triggering of the NLRP3 inflammasome results in the secretion of IL-1β, which is a key proinflammatory cytokine (Abrams et al., 2010; Meunier et al., 2012; Sandberg et al., 2012; Sun et al., 2013; Yang et al., 2012). Inflammasomes are multiprotein complexes that act as a major mediator for inflammatory responses. Among the various inflammasomes, NLRP3 inflammasomes are being the most studied and their activation has been linked to exposure of the biological system to nanomaterials of various compositions. For instance, double-walled carbon nanotubes enhanced the release of the proinflammatory cytokine IL-1β from human monocytes via the NLRP3 inflammasome activation pathway (Meunier et al., 2012). Production of IL-1β has also been observed upon incubation of human monocytes with silver nanoparticles, and the cytokine release was enhanced upon reducing the size of the particles (Yang et al., 2012). It was found that the silver nanoparticles induced inflammasome formation that triggered the release of the IL-1β.

3.4.2 Route of administration

3.4.2.1 Intravenous route

In general, parenteral administration is associated with a stronger immune response than oral administration, may be due to the lower bioavailability from the oral route, in contrast to the readily available immune cells to interact with the nanoparticles administered via the parenteral routes. Poly(D,L-lactide-*co*-glycolide) (PLGA) particles loaded with pertussis toxoid and filamentous haemagglutinin were able to induce potent T cell and antibody response to a higher extent when administered parenterally, as compared to the oral immunization, and hence lower dose and less frequent administration were required (Conway et al., 2001). Nanoparticles introduced into the body via an intravenous (i.v.) route are exposed to a complex environment of blood cells and proteins immediately upon injection. Most immediately adsorb blood proteins on their surfaces. The adsorption of plasma proteins to nanoparticle surfaces, composition of the protein corona, and interactions with blood cells determine biodistribution and therapeutic efficacy of the nanoparticles and may also contribute to immunotoxicity (Aggarwal et al., 2009; Dobrovolskaia et al., 2008). Opsonization is considered to be one of the major barriers to nanoparticle stability and delivery in vivo. The most common components of the nanoparticle protein corona are immunoglobulins, complement proteins, albumin, apolipoprotein, and fibrinogen (Dobrovolskaia & McNeil, 2007). Attachment of immunoglobulins and complement to the surface of nanoparticles tags them for attack by the MPS (Aggarwal et al., 2009). Blood cells exposed to certain nanoparticles may produce cytokines, but the mechanisms of cytokine induction are poorly understood.

3.4.2.2 Subcutaneous and dermal routes

Most nanoparticles do not cross intact skin barriers but can be engineered for dermal or transdermal delivery. Skin is an immunologically active site rich in immune cells such as the epidermal Langerhans' cells and dermal dendritic cells. This is why the delivery of nanoparticles via skin can initiate an inflammatory response. Several studies have demonstrated that small (<50 nm) nanoparticles administered subcutaneously distribute through lymphatic drainage into draining lymph nodes where they stimulate antigen-presenting cells and lymphocytes (Manolova et al., 2008; Reddy et al., 2007). Lymphatic drainage is thought to promote an adaptive immune response through several mechanisms involving local complement activation and stimulation of T-cells (Manolova et al., 2008; Reddy et al., 2007). Subcutaneous administration of PLGA nanoparticles loaded with antigens (tyrosinase-related protein 2 and 7-acyl lipid A) in mice activated dendritic cells and transmitted the immune response to the draining lymph nodes and spleen, as demonstrated by the secretion of IFN-γ at lymph nodes and spleen (Hamdy et al., 2008). The levels of the proinflammatory cytokines in the tumor tissues of the treated mice (bearing melanoma B16 tumors) were higher than in the control group (mice immunized with empty nanoparticles). The route of administration not only influences the extent of the immune response, but also the type of response. Intraperitoneal and intramuscular administration of pertussis toxoid and filamentous haemagglutinin in PLGA microparticles resulted in T_H1 response, whereas parenteral and oral immunization of the antigens in solution or loaded into PLGA nanoparticles resulted in T_H2 or mixed T_H1/T_H2 responses (Conway et al., 2001). The size, surface area, availability of antigens in various formulations, and route of administration might explain this difference in responses. In this study, immune response following subcutaneous immunization was inferior to the other parenteral routes of administration (i.e., intraperitoneal and intramuscular).

3.4.2.3 Nasal and oral routes

Delivery of nanoparticles via nasal and oral routes brings them in contact with the mucosa-associated lymphoid tissues and again may cause interaction with the residing macrophages or lymphocytes with possibilities of subsequent transportation of cells or the immune products to the circulation and other body tissues. Singh et al. (2006) demonstrated that the intranasal administration of PLGA-*b*-poly(ε-caprolactone) nanoparticles loaded with diphtheria toxoid induced higher production of the IL-6 and IFN-γ, as compared to the intramuscular administration of the same nanoparticles. However, this difference cannot be generalized to other types of nanomaterials as it depends on the characteristics of the nanoparticles and the nature of the antigenic payloads (Conway et al., 2001; Kumar et al., 2003; Thomas et al., 2011). In addition, the site of administration and the type of the APCs that first present the antigen and the cytokine environment at the activation site can all contribute to the type and extent of immune response and to the profile of the induced cytokines (Conway et al., 2001; Florindo et al., 2009; Gajewski et al., 1991; Kumar et al., 2003; Morikawa et al., 1993).

3.4.2.4 Intraperitoneal

Some researchers consider this route for nanoparticle-mediated drug delivery into tumors and it has been utilized for the treatment of other diseases. However, peritonitis (inflammation in the peritoneum) due to stimulation and recruitment of immune cells as well as systemic distribution of the particles and related off-target toxicities are common concerns. Several studies have demonstrated that certain nanomaterials can distribute systemically and cause inflammation and cytokine responses upon intraperitoneal administration. For example, Liu et al. (2012) has reported that mesoporous hollow silica nanoparticles administered via the intraperitoneal route cause induction of proinflammatory cytokines (IL-1β, TNF-α), liver damage, and activation of Kupffer cells. Another study demonstrated that nanosized TiO_2 nanoparticles caused oxidative stress, neutrophil activation, and inflammation in the lungs 4 h after intraperitoneal administration to mice. Analysis of the bronchoalveolar fluid from these animals has also revealed high levels of inflammatory cytokines TNF-α, IL-1β, and macrophage inflammatory protein (MIP)-2, the functional homolog of the human chemokine IL-8. Elevated gene expression of TNF and IL-1β was also found in lung tissues of animals exposed to TiO_2 particles via the intraperitoneal route (Moon et al., 2010). Other examples of off-target toxicity associated with induction of inflammatory cytokine responses by nanomaterials administered via the intraperitoneal route include brain inflammation and activation of microglial cells by coadministration of nanosized TiO_2 particles and low levels of endotoxin (Shin et al., 2010) and allergic sensitization and lung inflammation caused by coadministration of TiO_2 nanoparticles and ovalbumin (Larsen et al., 2010).

Distribution of nanoparticles from the peritoneum to other compartments and across the blood-brain barrier is interesting. The mechanisms of such traffic are poorly understood, but this strategy is being explored for therapeutic applications. For example, intraperitoneal administration of a C60 fullerene derivative into mice 9 h after challenge with gram-negative bacteria reduced inflammatory cytokine levels and protected mice from bacterial meningitis (Tsao et al., 1999). Similarly, intraperitoneal administration of dendrimer antisense oligonucleotide conjugates reduced cytokine secretion associated with infection of Japanese encephalitis (Nazmi et al., 2010). Another application is vaccine delivery. For example, antigen-loaded solid lipid nanoparticles were efficient in eliciting T_H1 type immune responses and cytokines in mice upon intraperitoneal administration (Doroud et al., 2011).

3.4.3 Endocytic pathways

The endocytic pathway, surface decorating moieties on the nanoparticles, and engagement of specific cellular receptors in the endocytosis process dictate the immune response. Phagocytosis is a receptor-mediated endocytosis restricted to professional phagocytes (e.g., macrophages, dendritic cells, platelets). There are four main phagocytic routes, mannose-receptor (Mr)-, complement receptor (CR)-, Fcγ receptor (FcγR), and scavenger receptor (SR)-mediated phagocytosis. Mannose, complement proteins, and immunoglobulins are opsonins targeting the Mr, CR, and FcγR routes, respectively (Aderem & Underhill, 1999). SRs are thought to react with negatively charged surfaces (Aderem & Underhill, 1999). Phagocytic cells can also utilize other routes to engulf and eliminate foreign materials. Some of these pathways are receptor-independent and include various forms of pinocytosis: macropinocytosis, clathrin-dependent, caveolin-dependent, and clathrin/caveolin-independent pinocytosis. In addition to phagocytic receptors, immune cells utilize many other surface and transmembrane proteins to sense and endocytose foreign materials. One type of such receptor is Toll-like receptor (TLR). TLRs are pattern recognition receptors that can either be associated with the membrane surfaces (e.g., TLRs 1, 2, 5, 4, and 6) or localized into the endosomes (e.g., TLRs 3, 7, 8, and 9). Each of these receptors can act alone or in cooperation with other members of this protein family to effectively recognize so-called pathogen-associated molecular patterns (PAMP). Examples of common PAMPs are bacterial lipoproteins, lipopolysaccharides, unmethylated cytosine-phosphate-guanine (CpG) motifs, and single- and double-stranded RNA (Iwasaki & Medzhitov, 2004; Pasare & Medzhitov, 2005). Activation of TLRs by their respective PAMPs results in the production of various cytokines, initiates inflammation, and coordinates cellular and humoral immunity (Pasare & Medzhitov, 2005; Tao et al., 2011). There are also other components of the immune system that regulate the immune response, such as cytoplasmic immunoreceptors (e.g., retinoid inducible gene-1 protein, nucleotide binding oligomerization domain (NOD)-like receptors (NLR), and retinoic acid-inducible gene (RIG)-like receptors) (Bortoluci & Medzhitov, 2010). Activation of these receptors initiates receptor-linked intracellular signaling pathways (e.g., nuclear factor-kappaB (NF-κB), interferon responsive factors, activating protein-1 (AP-1), interleukin-1 receptor-associated kinase, etc.) (Tao et al., 2011; Waes, 2007).

Various surface functionalization strategies have been undertaken to create nanoparticles with "pathogen-like" surface properties. For example, it has been demonstrated that nanoparticles can be engineered to target specific receptors (e.g., Mr-mediated phagocytosis) and induce cytokine responses by introducing mannosylated chitosan residues onto their surface (Kim et al., 2006). In another study, di-mannose and galactose, employed to modify the surface of polyanhydride nanoparticles, resulted in an increase in mannose receptor expression on the surface of alveolar macrophages, which was accompanied by an increased uptake of the particles (presumably through Mr-mediated phagocytosis). Binding to the receptors initiated a downstream signaling pathway that ends up with the production of proinflammatory cytokines (IL-1β, IL-6, and TNF-α), mainly through the activation of NF-κB. The production of the cytokines was higher for the targeted nanoparticles than for the nontargeted ones (Chavez-Santoscoy et al., 2012). Likewise, "grafting" the particle surface with C-type lectins was shown to increase their uptake into bone marrow-derived dendritic cells and induce inflammatory cytokine secretion (Carrillo-Conde et al., 2011). Another strategy involves the conjugation or encapsulation of specific PAMPs to nanoparticles. For example, it has been demonstrated that TLR ligands such as poly-IC, R848, and lipid A are effectively delivered into immune cells and act as adjuvants through the induction of cytokine secretion (Hamdy et al., 2007, 2008; Tacken et al., 2011). All these strategies are employed to generate deliberate cytokine responses to improve vaccine efficacy. However, nanoparticles unintended to be immunostimulatory (not designed to be vaccine adjuvants), but inducing cytokine responses, do not carry mannose or other ligands that would target the proinflammatory pathways. The mechanism of cytokine induction by this category of nanoparticles is less clear. For example, a study has shown that polyacrylic acid (PAA)-conjugated gold nanoparticles interact with the integrin receptor Mac-1 and induce secretion of inflammatory cytokines through a mechanism dependent on the binding and unfolding of fibrinogen (Deng et al., 2011). Interestingly, not all particles capable of binding plasma fibrinogen shared this property (Deng et al., 2011). It was proposed that activation of the Mac-1 receptors increases NF-κB activity by increasing the degradation of IκB, which allow the translocation of NF-κB into the nucleus and upregulate the expression of the proinflammatory genes. The fibrinogen-bound PAA-gold nanoparticles induced the release of IL-8 and TNF-α, although fibrinogen and PAA-gold nanoparticles could not induce the release of these cytokines. Inhibition of the NF-κB pathway reduced the release of these cytokines.

3.4.4 The role of the nanocarriers: physicochemical characteristics

The extent of opsonization, destabilization, and clearance depends mainly on the nanoparticle characteristics (Elsabahy & Wooley, 2012a). The composition of the nanoparticle, the size, charge, morphology, and most importantly, surface chemistry, dictate the toxicity and immune response induced by nanoparticles. The ability of nanoparticles to move into specific regions (e.g., lymphoid tissues) and to activate APCs greatly affects their immunomodulatory effects. Hence, it can be seen how the selective uptake and biodistribution of nanoparticles can greatly affect their immunogenicity. The stronger the interaction between the nanoparticle and cells, the higher the expected immune response. Hence, it is expected that cationic carriers administered via certain routes (e.g., subcutaneous or intradermal) will induce higher immunotoxicity and serve as better adjuvants (i.e., materials not antigenic per se but capable of enhancing the immune response to the antigen). Cationic liposomes were shown to induce the expression of T_H1 cytokines, most notably TNF-α, IFN-g, and IL-12, which are associated with tumor static effects (Cui et al., 2005). Cytokine induction was reported for other (noncationic) nanomaterials as well. For instance, exposure of dendritic cells to zinc oxide nanoparticles with negative zeta potentials (-31 to -36 mV) upregulated the expression of CD80 and CD86 and stimulated the release of proinflammatory cytokines (IL-6 and TNF-α), although there was no observable cytotoxic effects (Heng et al., 2011). CD80 and CD86 are proteins that can be found on activated B cells, monocytes, dendritic cells, and macrophages that work as costimulators for T cells activation (i.e., acting as ligands for proteins on T cell surface), and they are also well-known markers for dendritic cells activation and maturation.

3.4.4.1 Size

It has been reviewed previously in detail how the size of nanoparticles can determine their cellular uptake, intracellular trafficking pathways, biodistribution, and in vivo fate (Elsabahy & Wooley, 2012a; Iversen et al., 2011).

It has been generally found that the strength and type of immune response depend also on the size of the nanoparticles (Dobrovolskaia & McNeil, 2007; Dobrovolskaia et al., 2009; Hussain et al., 2012; Zolnik et al., 2010). Although it is still controversial, it has been reported several times that the nanometer-sized particles are more toxic than micrometer-sized particles, probably due to the increased surface-to-volume ratio (Singh et al., 2006). Hussain et al. have found that even small differences in the size of the particles can cause significant changes in the inflammatory responses. The immunotoxicity of carbon black and TiO_2 particles with average sizes of (13, 21, and 95 nm) and (15 and 25−75 nm), respectively, was tested at concentrations that are not cytotoxic to cells. The smallest nanoparticles of both types resulted in the highest induction of the GM-CSF cytokine (Hussain et al., 2009). The same study demonstrated also a dose- and cellular uptake-dependent induction of the inflammatory cytokine.

It has been demonstrated that the size of a nanomaterial affects both the type and the strength of the immune response to an antigen. For example, in an interesting study examining the effect of particle size on immune response, nanometer and micrometer (220, 500, and 1200 nm) RNA/protamine particles were utilized (Rettig et al., 2010). It was concluded that the smaller particles elicited viral-like responses by triggering the release of IFN-α, whereas the larger particles developed bacterial-like immune responses and induced the release of TNF-α, whereas neither of the nanoparticle components (RNA or protamine) could increase the level of any of the tested cytokines (IFN-α and TNF-α) in human peripheral blood mononuclear cells. It was suggested that the immune system distinguishes the size of the particles associated with the antigen (i.e., single-stranded RNA) to trigger antiviral and antibacterial/antifungal immune responses for the nano- and micro-sized particles, respectively. In other studies, it was observed that only small nanoparticles (about 50 nm) conjugated to a model antigen could induce T_H1 response, whereas antigen conjugates to larger particles tend to promote a T_H2 response (Fifis et al., 2004; Minigo et al., 2007; Mottram et al., 2007).

3.4.4.2 Shape and hydrophobicity

The effect of the shape of zinc oxide nanoparticles (spherical *vs.* sheet) of approximately similar specific surface area was studied. Although the higher cellular association of the spherical particles, there were no significant differences in the generation of the reactive oxygen species and in stimulating the secretion of proinflammatory cytokines (IL-6 and TNF-α) (Heng et al., 2011).

3.4.4.3 Composition and surface modifications

The effects of surface modification on the inflammatory effects of silica nanoparticles (30–1000 nm) have been studied by Morishige et al. both in vitro and in vivo (Morishige et al., 2012).

3.4.5 The contribution of the payloads

The cargo, not only the nanoparticle carrier composition, is of great importance. Several examples will be given in this section to emphasize the effect of the payload on the immunotoxicity of nanoparticles and will include nucleic acids and taxanes.

The administration of lipoplexes of pDNA or antisense oligonucleotides is usually associated with toxicity. Cationic lipoplexes [composed of 1,2-dioleoyl-3-trimethylammonium propane (DOTAP), cholesterol, protamine, and plasmid DNA (pDNA)] stimulated the expression of CD80/CD86 on dendritic cells and induced the release of TNF-α (Cui et al., 2005). It was concluded that both DNA and the cationic lipid (DOTAP) are required for full immunostimulation. The immunostimulatory sequences in the plasmid or smaller DNA structures (i.e., bacterial CpG motifs) can activate the immune system via the endosomal TLR9 (Rottembourg et al., 2010; Yoshida et al., 2009). The immune stimulation triggers the proliferation of the B cells and natural killer cells and the release of inflammatory cytokines (e.g., IFN-γ, IFN-α/β, IL-6, IL-12, GM-CSF, and TNF-α), which may lead to serious local and systemic inflammatory reactions (Karikó et al., 2004; Tan et al., 1999). It has been reported in clinical and preclinical studies that the administration of pDNA lipoplexes results in mild "flu-like" inflammatory syndrome in humans and increased levels of inflammatory cells and cytokines within the lungs of mice (Alton et al., 1999; Hyde et al., 2008; Ruiz et al., 2001). It is commonly observed that the DNA lipoplexes induce the secretion of inflammatory cytokines by T_H1 cells in a CpG-dependent manner (Freimark et al., 1998; Scheule et al., 1997) and this immunostimulation is usually associated with a reduction of gene expression in a dose-dependent manner (Hyde et al., 2008; Yew et al., 1999). Although this opens up the possibility of taking advantage of immunostimulatory effects of CpG motifs for vaccination, it might complicate the situation and may result in uncontrollable adverse reactions. In addition, there will be burdensome to the use of these vehicles as platforms for other biomedical delivery applications where immunostimulation is not desirable.

The systemic administration of RNA is often associated with immune stimulation both in vitro and in vivo, predominantly due to the interaction with TLRs 3, 7, and/or 8, and sometimes due to recognition by other immunoreceptors that recognize RNA and subsequently release proinflammatory cytokines (Judge et al., 2009; Semple et al., 2010). When formulated with lipids, RNA can trigger both the lipid- and RNA-sensing TLRs and cytoplasmic immunoreceptors (Judge & MacLachlan, 2008; Judge et al., 2006; Kim et al., 2007; Morrissey et al., 2005; Tao et al., 2011). As with DNA, the use of cationic lipids for siRNA delivery may result in inflammation and anaphylactic reactions (Abrams et al., 2010; Judge & MacLachlan, 2008; Sepp-Lorenzino & Ruddy, 2008). It has been reported that the systemic administration of lipid siRNA complexes triggers the release of proinflammatory cytokines and enhances the level of serum transaminases in mice at high doses (Abrams et al., 2010; Judge et al., 2005; Kim et al., 2007; Zimmermann et al., 2006). Examples of the cytokines that are usually induced upon systemic administration of siRNA include IL-1α, IL1-β, IL-6, IL-10, IL-12, keratinocyte-derived cytokine, TNF-α, IFN-α, IFN-γ, and MCP-1 (Abrams et al., 2010; Judge et al., 2005, 2006; Tao et al., 2011).

Immune responses to chemotherapeutic agents are also well established and were reported to contribute significantly to their anticancer activity (Zitvogel et al., 2008). For instance, taxanes are mitotic inhibitors that include paclitaxel and docetaxel. Their anticancer activity is achieved through binding to tubulins and inhibition of cell mitosis at the G2/M phase through stabilization of the microtubules, which triggers apoptosis (Yeung et al., 1999). However, the immunostimulation induced by taxanes contributes significantly to their anticancer activity (Javeed et al., 2009). It has been reported several times that the biological and immunostimulatory effects of taxanes are similar to those of lipopolysaccharides (bacterial components that elicit a strong immune response) (Byrd-Leifer et al., 2001; Javeed et al., 2009). Taxanes activate macrophages to initiate cytotoxicity against tumor cells. Activated macrophages also secrete cytokines (e.g., IL-1β, IL-8, IL-12, GM-CSF, and TNF-α), which in turn stimulate the cytotoxic lymphocytes and natural killer cells against cancer cells (tumoricidal activity) (Chan & Yang, 2000; Javeed et al., 2009).

3.5 Mechanisms of nanoparticle immunotoxicity

The exact mechanism of nanoparticle immunotoxicity and correlation with the endocytic pathways have not been clarified yet, due to the biological variability and dependence of the results on the exact composition of nanomaterials, cell type, cell cycle, animal model, disease status, etc. In addition, most of the studies utilize the various markers to predict the possible immunomodulatory effects of nanomaterials, rather than investigating the exact mechanisms beyond the immunotoxic effects and/or the differences in immune responses to nanoparticles of different size, shape, surface chemistry, and composition. Sometimes, the induction of both proinflammatory cytokines (e.g., IL-6 and TNF-α) and antiinflammatory cytokines (e.g., IL-10) due to unregulated innate immune response (i.e., cytokine storm) makes it harder to understand the underlying mechanisms of immunotoxicity (Stebbings et al., 2007; Suntharalingam et al., 2006). Dissection of the mechanism(s) of the proinflammatory response is often complicated by the presence of endotoxin in the nanoparticle formulations. Such contamination is common (Jones & Grainger, 2009), undesirable, and often overlooked. Removal of endotoxin from nanoparticles has been shown to eliminate cytokine response and fever reactions (Dobrovolskaia et al., 2010; Vallhov et al., 2006). Of interest is the increasing data demonstrating that some nanoparticles per se do not induce cytokine response but significantly enhance a cytokine response initiated by low concentrations of endotoxin. In some cases, the mechanism involves the NLR3 inflammasome (Hamilton et al., 2009; Reisetter et al., 2011). For example, fibrous, TiO_2 nanoparticles did not induce cytokines, but when these particles were combined with low, unreactive amounts of endotoxin they resulted in a strong induction of cytokines of the IL-1 family (IL-1β, IL18, IL33) through a cathepsin B-mediated mechanism (Hamilton et al., 2009). Cytokine storms and exaggeration of inflammatory reactions to endotoxin were also reported for several environmental nanoparticles (Fuhrmann et al., 2012; Hawkins et al., 2008; Shi et al., 2011). Another common culprit in undesired cytokine induction by engineered nanomaterials is chemical impurities (e.g., synthesis by-products and metal catalysts). For example, early studies on carbon nanotubes demonstrated that these particles can induce proinflammatory cytokine responses (Shvedova et al., 2005), but when these same particles were purified from iron contaminants, they were later shown to be non-immunostimulatory and did not induce cytokines (Murray et al., 2009; Pulskamp et al., 2007). Although all these complications in studying the mechanisms of immunotoxicity, mechanisms that have been mostly involved in the induction of cytokines release due to treatment of cells or animals with nanomaterials will be briefly discussed in this section.

Recognition of PAMPs derived from various pathogens by TLRs and/or cytoplasmic immunoreceptors (e.g., retinoid inducible gene-1) in the various immune cells stimulates the innate immune response and initiates signaling pathways that activate the transcription factor NF-κB and other pathways (e.g., p38/AP1, PI3K, and interferon regulatory factor 3/5/7), which lead to the production of proinflammatory cytokines (Cui et al., 2005; Tao et al., 2011). Activation of NF-κB can occur via various mediators, such as proinflammatory cytokines, TLRs, reactive oxygen species, and others (Tao et al., 2011; Waes, 2007). The NF-κB controls the expression of several proinflammatory cytokines and upregulation of costimulatory molecules on dendritic cells, which are required for activation of T cells. In addition, it plays a pivotal role in coordinating innate and adaptive immunity (Blackwell & Christman, 1997; Kawai & Akira, 2007; Lawrence, 2009). This transcription factor presents in the cytoplasmic inactive form that is bound to inhibitory proteins called IκBs. Activation of NF-κB upon cell stimulation, which can occur through multiple pathways, phosphorylates and degrades the IκBs, where the free NF-κB translocates from the cytoplasm to the nucleus to control the transcription of several cytokines. The detailed mechanisms of the NF-κB activation and subsequent induction of secreting inflammatory cytokines have been reviewed elsewhere (Blackwell & Christman, 1997; Kawai & Akira, 2007; Lawrence, 2009). Activation of TLRs can occur through the NF-κB and mitogen-activated protein kinases (MAPKs) and stimulate the production of proinflammatory cytokines, maturation of dendritic cells, and expression of costimulatory molecules (e.g., CD80 and CD86) on their surfaces (Cui et al., 2005; Heng et al., 2011). The activated dendritic cells can then migrate to the local lymphoid tissues for antigen presentation. It was reported in one study that cationic liposomes (DOTAP) stimulated the expression of CD80 and CD86 on dendritic cells without inducing the release of TNF-α, due to the NF-κB independent pathway (Cui et al., 2005). Another study suggested the presence of multiple pathways for induction of toxicities and release of cytokines. In this study, pretreatment with inhibitors of multiple pathways (e.g., PI3K, mTOR, p38/AP1, and NF-κB) partially inhibited the release of cytokines induced by siRNA-lipid nanoparticles (Tao et al., 2011).

Recognition of immunostimulatory lipids by TLR2 and TLR4 on the cell surface of macrophages and other cells initiates proinflammatory transcriptional programs, including induction of several cytokines (Takeda et al., 2003). In one study, several cytokines (IL-1α, IL-1β, IL-6, KC, IL-10, IFN-γ, and TNF-α) were released in the plasma of mice treated with lipid nanoparticles, and inflammatory reactions were mainly attributed to the lipid components (Abrams et al., 2010). The mice treated with the same lipid (cationic lipid, CLinDMA), but formulated in emulsion, caused a similar cytokine release response in mice. Pretreatment with an intraperitoneal injection of dexamethasone (glucocorticoid receptor agonist) inhibited the cytokine release and inflammation in multiple tissues in a dose-dependent manner. Usually, activation of this cytoplasmic nuclear hormone receptor inhibits the transcriptional activity of NF-κB and can inhibit multiple pathways of inflammatory reactions (Kawai & Akira, 2007; Morand, 2007; Moynagh, 2003).

In several other studies, it was reported that both lipids and nucleic acids are required for immunostimulation, which can be explained by several hypotheses (Cui et al., 2005). One of the possible reasons is that cationic complexes enhance the cellular uptake of DNA/RNA. For instance, induction of cytokines and cellular influx in the lung airway were observed following intratracheal administration of an *N*-[1-(2−3-dioleyloxy)propyl]-*N,N,N*-trimethylammonium chloride/cholesterol/plasmid positively charged complexes in mice (Freimark et al., 1998). The cytokine release was enhanced by complexing the plasmid to the cationic lipid. Another hypothesis is that the synergistic effect is due to separate responses to the nucleic acid and lipid, which results in two different sets of cytokines. In addition, the released cytokines due to treatment with one component may induce the secretion of other cytokines. A potential mechanism could also be the protection afforded by the electrostatic complexation against enzymatic degradation, which sustains the immunostimulatory effect of nucleic acids. Furthermore, the cationic carriers facilitate the delivery of DNA/RNA to local lymphoid tissues, where they can activate APCs.

Nanoparticles may also generate large quantities of reactive oxygen species that can trigger the release of proinflammatory cytokines through the activation of NF-κB (Heng et al., 2011; Morishige et al., 2012). The production of reactive oxygen species might be higher for nanoparticles than microparticles due to the enhanced surface area and surface reactivity (Morishige et al., 2012). Carbon black, TiO_2 nanoparticles induced the release of cytokines in the bronchial epithelial cell line via oxidative stress (Hussain et al., 2009; Val et al., 2009). The inflammatory effect and release of cytokines were inhibited by catalase, an enzyme that protects against oxidative stress by catalyzing the decomposition of hydrogen peroxide into oxygen and water. Crystalline silica nanoparticles generated reactive oxygen species that triggered TNF-receptors, which activated the cellular NF-κB transcription factor and resulted in an inflammatory response (Beyerle et al., 2010).

3.6 Relationship between cytokines and adverse reactions

Modification of the immune system functions can lead to various consequences ranging from mild adverse reactions to serious and fatal immune complications. Lymphocyte proliferation in response to stimulation by an antigen or mitogen is a direct reflection of cellular immunity and is usually associated with the production of antibodies or cytokines (Mottram et al., 2007). In vitro and in vivo studies are confirming that nanomaterials can interact with the immune system and stimulate the production of proinflammatory cytokines, which are capable of recruiting inflammatory cells including basophils, macrophages, dendritic cells, T cells, neutrophils, and eosinophils (Benjamini et al., 2000). The immune response against the nanoparticles or their payloads may be beneficial or detrimental depending on the intended use of the given nanoformulation, its mode of action, and the route of administration (Zolnik et al., 2010). For example, inflammation and granuloma formation have been observed in tissues exposed to unfunctionalized multiwalled carbon nanotubes (Witzmann & Monteiro-Riviere, 2006).

Cytokines play an important role in orchestrating and controlling the inflammatory process and their continual presence or excessive production can result in serious adverse reactions that can be life-threatening. They are also involved in important processes, such as fetal recognition, placental development, and regulation of gene expression during organogenesis (Batista-Duharte et al., 2011). They are directly or indirectly involved in the pathogenesis of several immune-mediated disorders and their levels are usually altered in patients with cancers, cardiovascular diseases, inflammatory diseases (e.g., rheumatoid arthritis), and infectious diseases (e.g., hepatitis) (Khan et al., 2009; Kidd, 2003; Kokkonen et al., 2010; Shiraki et al., 2011; Tashiro et al., 1997; Vistnes et al., 2010). For instance, it was found that the levels of several cytokines (IL-1β, IL-2, IL-4, IL-6, IL-7, IL-10, IL-12, TNF, IFN-g, GM-CSF, G-CSF, MCP-1, MIP-1a, Eotaxin) were significantly higher in individuals before disease onset of rheumatoid arthritis than in control subjects and further increased after the disease (Kokkonen et al., 2010).

Cytokines can mediate both local and systemic inflammatory responses, and they can also be distributed throughout the circulation to various sites of activity. The resulting immune system derangement can lead to an increased incidence of autoimmune, allergic, and even neoplastic diseases. Some cytokines, such as IL-1, IL-2, IL-6, TNF, transforming growth factor (TGF)-β, and IFNs, are also involved in modulating the expression of several P450 isoforms (i.e., modification of hepatic metabolism) (Batista-Duharte et al., 2011). Some of these circulating cytokines can enter some organs through fenestrated capillaries where they induce the production of prostaglandins (PG), such as PGE2, a centrally controlled mediator of fever (Batista-Duharte et al., 2011). The role of cytokines in the immunotoxicity of small and macromolecules has been established, and molecular mechanisms are well understood. Studies connecting cytokines to specific toxicities associated with the use of engineered nanomaterials have been reported, but the molecular mechanisms have yet to be defined. For example, an interesting study was performed to confirm the role of cytokines in inducing toxicities. Systemic administration of siRNA-encapsulated lipid nanoparticles induced the release of several cytokines such as TNF-α, IL-6, IFN-γ, and MCP-1 (Tao et al., 2011). These cytokines were correlated with toxicity. Mild alleviation of the toxic responses was observed when the toxicity of the nanoparticles was re-evaluated in mouse lines deficient in one of these cytokines. Hence, it can be concluded that knocking down one or some of these cytokines is not enough to prevent the toxicity associated with the administration of the siRNA-loaded nanoparticles. Another recent study linked induction of IL-8 to dermal toxicity induced by iron oxide nanoparticles (Murray et al., 2013) and to pulmonary toxicity associated with the in vivo use of various metal oxide nanomaterials (Cho et al., 2012). Similarly, induction of acute inflammatory cytokines (IL-1, TNF-α, IL-6, IL-8, etc.) was linked to nephrotoxicity associated with the in vivo use of TiO_2 nanoparticles (Gui et al., 2011). As the analysis of cytokine levels in the blood is more accessible than the analysis of specific pulmonary, dermal, and nephrotoxicity markers, ex vivo analysis of cytokines may contribute to the identification and understanding of the mechanisms of these toxicities.

3.7 Evaluation of nanoparticle immunotoxicity

There are a variety of methods for evaluating the immunotoxicity of nanomaterials both in vitro and in vivo, with each technique subject to specific limitations (Dobrovolskaia et al., 2009). According to the practical strategies suggested during the National Cancer Institute's Nanoparticle Immunotoxicity Workshop, it is essential to test for endotoxin contamination before studying the immunotoxicity of nanomaterials in vitro and/or in vivo (Dobrovolskaia et al., 2009). Recently, a book that outlines various approaches that can be pursued for testing the safety of nanomaterials including sterility (endotoxin and microbial contamination) and immunological assays (hemolytic and thrombogenic properties, complement activation, uptake by macrophages, and cellular chemotaxis) became available (McNeil, 2011). The various assays available to test the toxicity of nanomaterials have also been reviewed elsewhere (Arora et al., 2012; Kroll et al., 2009; Marquis et al., 2009; Stone et al., 2009).

Most cytokines have a broad spectrum of biological activity on a wide variety of cells and are involved in hematopoiesis and recruitment of cells for host defense. Quantifying the levels of specific cytokines in cells, animals, or patients treated with nanoparticles is of particular importance because variation in the levels may provide an insight into the mechanisms of immunomodulation. Understanding the underlying mechanisms that induce the secretion of cytokines and the associated adverse reactions is essential in the design of safe nanoparticulates. In addition, cytokines act as mediators of various adverse reactions and provide insight into the prognosis of several diseases. They are also commonly used as therapeutics, for instance, for cancer immunotherapy (Kutzler & Weiner, 2008; Mahvi et al., 2007). The use of dynamic assays that include the assessment of the immune response to nanoparticles via simultaneous measurements of various cytokines can offer significant advantages, although it may be difficult to predict a clinically relevant response. These levels are often compared to the levels in untreated subjects and can also be compared to the normal physiological range for the cytokine of interest, provided such data are available (Chapman et al., 2010).

3.7.1 Multiplexing principles and complications

3.7.1.1 Principles

Even in the absence of an acute cellular or in vivo toxicity, elevated cytokines may induce an immune response and result in long-term undesirable immunotoxicity by affecting immune cell function. Hence, it is important to measure cytokines while establishing the safety profiles of engineered nanomaterials. There are various techniques for quantitative measurements of cytokines, proteins, and various inflammatory mediators, with varying degrees of specificity and accuracy. One of the most common and earliest approaches is the enzyme-linked immunosorbent assay (ELISA). More recently, multiplex arrays gained popularity due to the reduced cost per single cytokine and often reduced sample volume (Khan et al., 2009; Leng et al., 2008). There are several available technologies that utilize capture antibodies immobilized on microspheres, the most common being the cytometric bead assay, coupled particle light scattering, and multianalyte profiling (xMAP) technology (Bernhard et al., 2011; Elshal & McCoy, 2006). This review will not detail the comprehensive procedures or types of these immunoassays but will highlight the key features of the multiplex arrays as a new strategy for evaluating a large number of biomolecules (up to 100) in a few microliters (e.g., as low as 12 μL of serum or plasma samples) in a single sample with high sensitivity and accuracy.

The multiplex assay is a modified ELISA assay that has been adapted to measure multiple cytokines in the same sample simultaneously by utilizing several techniques, most commonly flow cytometric technology. It is less time consuming and labor-intensive and requires lower sample volume and provides higher throughput analysis than traditional ELISA assays. The assay is based on the incubation of samples from various sources (plasma, serum, tissue culture supernatant, cell or tissue lysates, lavage samples, or other matrices) that contain cytokines or other inflammatory mediators with a mixture of beads (Fig. 3.5). Each bead is coated with specific detection antibodies for every cytokine. The incubation is followed by a series of washes to remove the unbound cytokines. Biotinylated-antibodies are then added to bind to the cytokine-detection antibody complex (on a secondary site of the cytokine), which is conjugated onto the bead to form a sandwich-like complex. The detection products are then formed by the addition of a reporter molecule (e.g., streptavidin-phycoerythrin conjugate) that has a high binding affinity to the biotin (in the biotinylated antibody) and serves at the same time as a reporter or fluorescent indicator (correlated to cytokine concentration). The microscopic beads themselves are then recognized based on their chromogenic or fluorescence pattern (having unique color codes or spectral properties that correlate with the cytokine type) during the analysis (Fig. 3.5). Although methods of cell stimulation are more or less optimized and harmonized, evaluation of cytokine levels is still subjective and usually conducted based on convenience, affordability, and instrument availability in each individual laboratory. This emphasizes the need for greater harmonization and standardization of cytokine evaluation platforms.

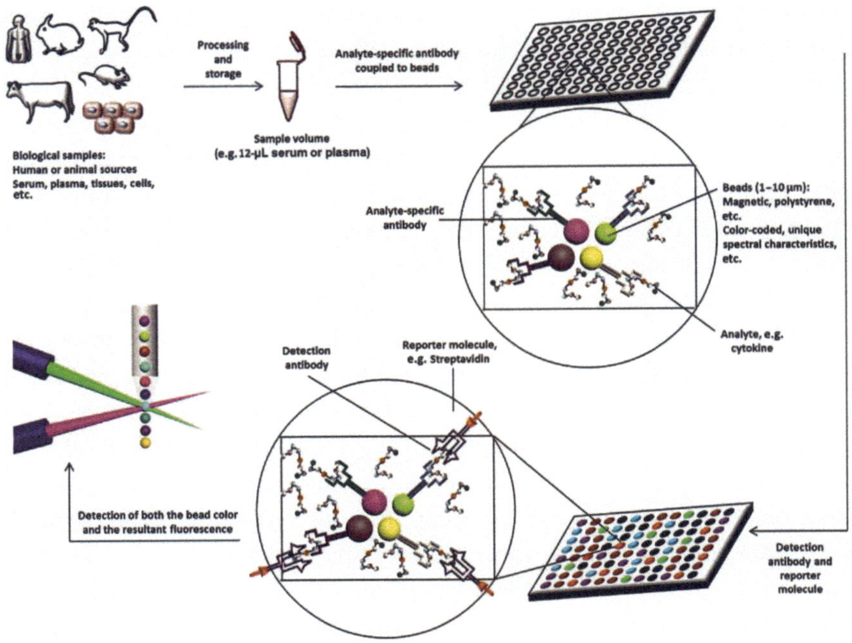

Figure 3.5 Schematic representation of the steps of multiplex assay for the simultaneous detection and measurements of cytokines in biological samples of various sources. Detailed procedures are not included in this schematic diagram and the detection methods (e.g., color code vs fluorescence, the use of various reporters, or the flow cytometric detection) vary depending on the specific instrument and kit utilized for the assay.

3.7.1.2 Complications

The common limitations of the multiplex arrays include signal "leach-over" between various analytes and the necessity of testing the same sample at multiple dilutions to "concentrate" some low abundance cytokines (e.g., IL4, IL-5) and dilute higher abundance cytokines (e.g., IL-8, TNF-α, IL1) to the assay range. Information on the expected serum levels of various cytokines is required for the proper dilution of samples. For instance, among 48 different cytokines analyzed in human serum, the mean values for most of the cytokines were <100 pg/mL (Chapman et al., 2010). However, some cytokines [e.g., IL-1β, G-CSF, and β-nerve growth factor (NGF)] had levels lower than the detection limit of the instruments (e.g., ~ 1.5 pg/mL for Bio-plex, Bio-Rad Laboratories, Inc., Hercules, CA), whereas platelet-derived growth factor (PDGF)-BB, regulated upon activation normal T-cell expressed and presumably secreted (RANTES) and stem cell growth factor (SCGF)-β concentrations were too high and required further dilutions (Chapman et al., 2010). Another hypothesis is that the antibody pair and the detection reagents need to be tuned to detect the cytokines that are either below or above the detection limits (i.e., these might be technique-related limitations). The multiplex arrays-based analyses are also extremely sensitive to the handling procedures and good laboratory practices (e.g., pipetting, consistency, use of standard operating procedures, validation, calibration, etc.).

Cytokines have short half-lives, which must be taken into consideration during analysis. Several cytokines have plasma half-lives ranging from minutes to a few hours [e.g., around 6–7 min for TNF-α (Beutler et al., 1985; Munoz et al., 1991)]. Hence, cytokines that can be detected in plasma over a long period of time suggest an intensive production. The timing is of particular importance for evaluating the levels of released cytokines. For instance, the release of 27 cytokines from corneal bilayers treated with nanoparticles was measured 1 h and 24 h after exposure to cobalt-chromium nanoparticles. Among the 27 cytokines, IL6, GM-CSF, growth regulated oncogene (GRO), MCP-1, and IL8 were significantly induced, but this was only observed at the 24 h time point (Sood et al., 2011). A general trend throughout the literature is that the levels of cytokines change significantly during the time course of the treatment with nanomaterials, both in vitro and in vivo. Hence, it is critical to compare samples that were collected at the same time, and stored, transported, and analyzed under identical conditions. In addition to the effect of timing, the possibility of interactions between nanoparticles and the secreted cytokines should also be considered. Adsorption of cytokines (e.g., GM-CSF, IL-6, and TNF-α) on various types of inorganic nanoparticles (e.g., carbon black and TiO_2 nanoparticles) has been observed in vitro, which might result in artifacts and misinterpretation of the data (Hussain et al., 2009; Kocbach et al., 2008; Val et al., 2009; Veranth et al., 2007). Other problems that could further complicate the assay and negatively affect the accuracy of the collected data include the presence of certain proteins in the analyzed samples, particularly the plentiful endogenous proteins in the blood, or the iron produced from blood hemolysis, which may interfere with the formation of cytokine–antibody complexes.

3.8 Controlling the immunotoxicity of nanomaterials

Proper design of nanomaterials has been always a subject of interest to improve their in vitro and in vivo characteristics, mainly to impart greater stability to their cargoes and to prolong blood circulation times to allow the accumulation at target sites, as well as greater safety. However, little impetus has been directed toward designing nanomaterials of low immunogenicity. When designing nanoparticles of low toxicity and immunogenicity, every component in the nanomaterial should be considered and systematic studies should be carried out to evaluate the effect of structural modifications on immunotoxicity. It is equally important to consider both the nanoparticle-forming material and the drug/payload (Fig. 3.6).

3.8.1 Nanoparticle-related factors

The first parameter to be considered in the design of nanoparticles is the shell thickness, density and type, and accessibility of any molecules used for surface decoration (e.g., targeting ligands, contrast agents). Functionalization of PLGA nanoparticles with thiol groups was tested to decrease interactions with opsonins and phagocytic cells and found to reduce protein adsorption, complement activation, and platelet activation of PLGA nanoparticles (Thasneem et al., 2011). Cationic nanoparticles are believed to be more

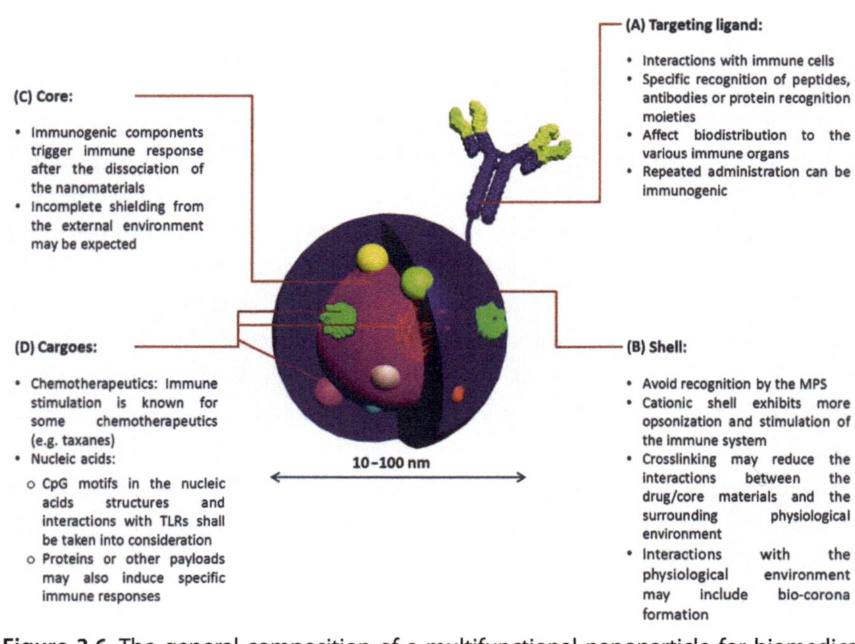

Figure 3.6 The general composition of a multifunctional nanoparticle for biomedical delivery applications. Some important considerations for the design of nanoparticles of low immunogenicity are illustrated with highlighting in the figure. The size of nanomaterials usually ranges from 10 to 100 nm.

toxic, rapidly cleared, and induce higher inflammatory reactions than their anionic or neutral counterparts. Encapsulation of therapeutics inside the nanocarrier is expected to reduce the immune response induced by the drug. Considering the approximate size of plasma proteins and constituents (~1–10 nm), it is desirable to keep the spacing between PEG chains as small as possible to minimize the interactions between the plasma components and the core material (Abrams et al., 2010; Meunier et al., 2012; Sandberg et al., 2012; Sun et al., 2013; Yang et al., 2012). Crosslinking the corona by biodegradable crosslinkers is also important to retain the spacing and avoid the dissociation and segregation of the PEG chains. Shell decoration with different moieties is necessary for the preparation of multifunctional nanocarriers. However, it is a prerequisite to keep the functionalization ratio as low as possible. In addition, the use of moieties of low immunogenicity (e.g., galactose instead of antibody for targeting) is recommended. Comprehensive studies to identify the critical parameters [e.g., PEG length and density (Fukukawa et al., 2008; Pressly et al., 2007; Sun et al., 1997)] that influence the toxicity and immunotoxicity of nanoparticles are required. In vitro studies to determine which blood components are involved in the destabilization/opsonization of nanoparticles are equally important for the rational design of nanoparticles. Polymer biodegradability and biocompatibility are essential for patient safety.

Careful selection of the ingredients of nanomaterials is critical in predicting the immune response upon in vivo administration. Indeed, Huang and coworkers have been systemically investigating the effect of the nanoparticle design on the immunotoxicity of nanoparticles designed for siRNA delivery. Targeted nanoparticles based on anisamide (ligand for sigma receptors overexpressed in some cancer cell lines)-PEGylated liposomes (DOTAP and cholesterol)-protamine-hyaluronic acid complexes (diameter of 115 nm and zeta-potential of 25 mV) were developed for the systemic delivery of siRNA (Chono et al., 2008). These nanoparticles showed low immunotoxicity in a dose range of 0.15–1.2 mg siRNA/kg in mice. On the contrary, another formulation that has the same composition but uses pDNA or calf thymus DNA instead of the hyaluronic acid had a narrower therapeutic index (e.g., a dose range of 0.15–0.45 mg/kg for the calf thymus DNA) (Li & Wallace, 2008; Wolfrum et al., 2007). The differences between the two formulations were the type of condensing materials that were employed to enhance the condensation of siRNA by cationic liposomes (DNA instead of hyaluronic acid). Intravenous injection of the siRNA formulated in both formulations in mice was tested, and proinflammatory cytokines (IL-6 and IL-12) levels in the serum of treated mice were measured 2-h after injection. The hyaluronic acid-based formulation induced lower immunotoxicity than the calf thymus or the pDNA-based nanoparticles, although both formulations showed similar characteristics and gene silencing activity. The lower immunotoxicity might be due to the removal of the foreign DNA and the CpG immunostimulatory sequences and also because hyaluronic acid is a biogenic compound that is widely distributed in human body fluids. Continuing on their work, nanoparticles built with a degradable calcium phosphate core were utilized instead of the nondegradable ones for the systemic delivery of siRNA and resulted in higher silencing activity in vitro and similar in vivo gene silencing. Importantly, they induced lower immunogenicity in mice as compared to the DNA/protamine-based nanoparticles (lower induction of IL-6 and IL-12 at higher doses) (Li et al., 2010).

3.8.2 Drug-related factors

Careful design of the drug itself can modulate the immunotoxicity of nanoparticles. For instance, while the injection of pDNA usually induces strong immune responses, designing plasmid structures that do not contain unmethylated CpG motifs could reduce the immunological reactions and enhance the transgene expression efficiency (Hyde et al., 2008). Surprisingly, even a single CpG motif in the DNA structure could elicit an inflammatory response. Methylation of pDNA has also been confirmed to significantly reduce the levels of inflammatory cytokines (Tan et al., 1999). Similarly, chemical modifications and sequence selection of other small nucleic acids (e.g., siRNA) can greatly modify/amend their immunotoxicity (Watts et al., 2008). It has been shown in one study that the immunostimulatory response of siRNA could be completely abolished, with no induction of cytokines (e.g., IFN-α and TNF), by designing chemically modified siRNA containing 2′-*O*-methyl modified nucleosides ($<20\%$) into one of the siRNA strands without affecting their gene-silencing activity, both in vitro and in vivo, whereas the unmodified siRNA induced the induction of cytokines and toxicity in the treated mice (Judge et al., 2006).

3.9 Conclusions

With the rapid and extensive research now underway into the design of novel nanomedicines, it is critical that attention be directed to their potential immunotoxicity. Evaluation of the immunotoxicity of nanomaterials, for example, by measuring the levels of cytokines or other immune indicators, is of particular importance for their clinical safety and for maximizing therapeutic benefits. Measuring the levels of proinflammatory cytokines and other inflammatory mediators and monitoring the balance of T_H1/T_H2 cytokines can be useful tools in evaluating nanoparticle immunotoxicity. Moreover, screening of a single reporter is inadequate; combinations of cytokine levels should be measured, due to the cytokine network influence on the immune system. Monitoring the levels of cytokines, in particular the proinflammatory ones, following administration of nanomaterials, appears to be an important tool for partially screening their immunomodulatory effects. High levels of cytokines, as compared to the untreated controls, are considered as biomarkers of nanoparticle immunotoxicity. The latter is usually associated with toxicity, adverse reactions, and lower therapeutic efficacy. Sometimes, treatment with antiinflammatory drugs might be useful in reducing the inflammatory effects associated with the administration of nanoparticles. Designing nanocarriers with biodegradable cores and coatings that are capable of shielding the core ingredients during circulation can minimize the immune response. Equally important is the design of the drug itself, for example via chemical modifications of nucleic acid (DNA/RNA) backbones to mask or remove immunostimulatory sequences. Further understanding of the underlying mechanisms of nanomaterial-mediated toxicities and inflammatory reactions, and the role of the various chemical mediators and ligands will secure the development of biocompatible and nonimmunogenic nanomaterials for a variety of biomedical delivery applications.

References

Abrams, M. T., Koser, M. L., Seitzer, J., Williams, S. C., Dipietro, M. A., Wang, W., Shaw, A. W., Mao, X., Jadhav, V., Davide, J. P., Burke, P. A., Sachs, A. B., Stirdivant, S. M., & Sepp-Lorenzino, L. (2010). Evaluation of efficacy, biodistribution, and inflammation for a potent siRNA nanoparticle: Effect of dexamethasone co-treatment. *Molecular Therapy*, *18*(1), 171–180. Available from https://doi.org/10.1038/mt.2009.208.

Aderem, A., & Underhill, D. M. (1999). Mechanisms of phagocytosis in macrophages. *Annual Review of Immunology*, *17*, 593–623. Available from https://doi.org/10.1146/annurev.immunol.17.1.593.

Aggarwal, P., Hall, J. B., McLeland, C. B., Dobrovolskaia, M. A., & McNeil, S. E. (2009). Nanoparticle interaction with plasma proteins as it relates to particle biodistribution, biocompatibility and therapeutic efficacy. *Advanced Drug Delivery Reviews*, *61*(6), 428–437. Available from https://doi.org/10.1016/j.addr.2009.03.009.

Alton, E. W. F. W., Stern, M., Farley, R., Jaffe, A., Chadwick, S. L., Phillips, J., Davies, J., Smith, S. N., Browning, J., Davies, M. G., Hodson, M. E., Durham, S. R., Li, D., Jeffery, P. K., Scallan, M., Balfour, R., Eastman, S. J., Cheng, S. H., Smith, A. E., & Geddes, D. M. (1999). Cationic lipid-mediated CFTR gene transfer to the lungs and nose of patients with cystic fibrosis: A double-blind placebo-controlled trial. *Lancet*, *353*(9157), 947–954. Available from https://doi.org/10.1016/S0140-6736(98)06532-5.

Arora, S., Rajwade, J. M., & Paknikar, K. M. (2012). Nanotoxicology and in vitro studies: The need of the hour. *Toxicology and Applied Pharmacology*, *258*(2), 151–165. Available from https://doi.org/10.1016/j.taap.2011.11.010.

Batista-Duharte, A., Lindblad, E. B., & Oviedo-Orta, E. (2011). Progress in understanding adjuvant immunotoxicity mechanisms. *Toxicology Letters*, *203*(2), 97–105. Available from https://doi.org/10.1016/j.toxlet.2011.03.001.

Bedi, D., Musacchio, T., Fagbohun, O. A., Gillespie, J. W., Deinnocentes, P., Bird, R. C., Bookbinder, L., Torchilin, V. P., & Petrenko, V. A. (2011). Delivery of siRNA into breast cancer cells via phage fusion protein-targeted liposomes. *Nanomedicine: Nanotechnology, Biology, and Medicine*, 7(3), 315–323. Available from https://doi.org/10.1016/j.nano.2010.10.004.

Benjamini, E., Coico, R., & Sunshine, G. (2000). *Immunology*. New York: John Wiley & Sons, Inc.

Bernhard, O. K., Mathias, R. A., Barnes, T. W., & Simpson, R. J. (2011). A fluorescent microsphere-based method for assay of multiple analytes in plasma. *Methods in Molecular Biology*, *728*, 195–206. Available from https://doi.org/10.1007/978-1-61779-068-3_12.

Beutler, B. A., Milsark, I. W., & Cerami, A. (1985). Cachectin/tumor necrosis factor: Production, distribution, and metabolic fate in vivo. *Journal of Immunology*, *135*(6), 3972–3977.

Beyerle, A., Irmler, M., Beckers, J., Kissel, T., & Stoeger, T. (2010). Toxicity pathway focused gene expression profiling of PEI-based polymers for pulmonary applications. *Molecular Pharmaceutics*, 7(3), 727–737. Available from https://doi.org/10.1021/mp900278x.

Black, C. A. (1999). Delayed type hypersensitivity: Current theories with an historic perspective. *Dermatology Online Journal*, *5*.

Blackwell, T. S., & Christman, J. W. (1997). The role of nuclear factor-κB in cytokine gene regulation. *American Journal of Respiratory Cell and Molecular Biology*, *17*(1), 3–9. Available from https://doi.org/10.1165/ajrcmb.17.1.f132.

Bortoluci, K. R., & Medzhitov, R. (2010). Control of infection by pyroptosis and autophagy: Role of TLR and NLR. *Cellular and Molecular Life Sciences*, *67*(10), 1643–1651. Available from https://doi.org/10.1007/s00018-010-0335-5.

Breslin, S. (2007). Cytokine-release syndrome: Overview and nursing implications. *Clinical Journal of Oncology Nursing*, *11*(1), 37–42.

Byrd-Leifer, C. A., Block, E. F., Takeda, K., Akira, S., & Ding, A. (2001). The role of MyD88 and TLR4 in the LPS-mimetic activity of Taxol. *European Journal of Immunology*, *31*(8), 2448–2457. Available from https://doi.org/10.1002/1521-4141(200108)31:8 < 2448::AID-IMMU2448 > 3.0.CO;2-N.

Carrillo-Conde, B., Song, E. H., Chavez-Santoscoy, A., Phanse, Y., Ramer-Tait, A. E., Pohl, N. L. B., Wannemuehler, M. J., Bellaire, B. H., & Narasimhan, B. (2011). Mannose-functionalized \pathogen-like\ polyanhydride nanoparticles target C-type lectin receptors on dendritic cells. *Molecular Pharmaceutics*, *8*(5), 1877–1886. Available from https://doi.org/10.1021/mp200213r.

Chan, O. T. M., & Yang, L. X. (2000). The immunological effects of taxanes. *Cancer Immunology Immunotherapy*, *49*(4–5), 181–185. Available from https://doi.org/10.1007/s002620000122.

Chang, C. (2010). The immune effects of naturally occurring and synthetic nanoparticles. *Journal of Autoimmunity*, *34*, 34234–34246.

Chapman, P., Reyes, C., & Gupta, V. (2010). Normal physiological levels of human cytokines using bio-plex ProTM cytokine assays. *Bio-Rad Tech Note*, 6029.

Chavez-Santoscoy, A. V., Roychoudhury, R., Pohl, N. L. B., Wannemuehler, M. J., Narasimhan, B., & Ramer-Tait, A. E. (2012). Tailoring the immune response by targeting C-type lectin receptors on alveolar macrophages using "pathogen-like" amphiphilic polyanhydride nanoparticles. *Biomaterials*, *33*(18), 4762–4772. Available from https://doi.org/10.1016/j.biomaterials.2012.03.027.

Cho, W. S., Duffin, R., Poland, C. A., Duschl, A., Oostingh, G. J., MacNee, W., Bradley, M., Megson, I. L., & Donaldson, K. (2012). Differential pro-inflammatory effects of metal oxide nanoparticles and their soluble ions in vitro and in vivo; Zinc and copper nanoparticles, but not their ions, recruit eosinophils to the lungs. *Nanotoxicology*, *6*(1), 22–35. Available from https://doi.org/10.3109/17435390.2011.552810.

Chono, S., Li, S. D., Conwell, C. C., & Huang, L. (2008). An efficient and low immunostimulatory nanoparticle formulation for systemic siRNA delivery to the tumor. *Journal of Controlled Release*, *131*(1), 64–69. Available from https://doi.org/10.1016/j.jconrel.2008.07.006.

Conway, M. A., Madrigal-Estebas, L., McClean, S., Brayden, D. J., & Mills, K. H. G. (2001). Protection against Bordetella pertussis infection following parenteral or oral immunization with antigens entrapped in biodegradable particles: Effect of formulation and route of immunization on induction of Th1 and Th2 cells. *Vaccine*, *19*(15–16), 1940–1950. Available from https://doi.org/10.1016/S0264-410X(00)00433-3.

Cubillos-Ruiz, J. R., Engle, X., Scarlett, U. K., Martinez, D., Barber, A., Elgueta, R., Wang, L., Nesbeth, Y., Durant, Y., Gewirtz, A. T., Sentman, C. L., Kedl, R., & Conejo-Garcia, J. R. (2009). Polyethylenimine-based siRNA nanocomplexes reprogram tumor-associated dendritic cells via TLR5 to elicit therapeutic antitumor immunity. *Journal of Clinical Investigation*, *119*(8), 2231–2244. Available from https://doi.org/10.1172/JCI37716.

Cui, Z., Han, S. J., Vangasseri, D. P., & Huang, L. (2005). Immunostimulation mechanism of LPD nanoparticle as a vaccine carrier. *Molecular Pharmaceutics*, *2*(1), 22–28. Available from https://doi.org/10.1021/mp049907k.

Davis, M. E., Zuckerman, J. E., Choi, C. H. J., Seligson, D., Tolcher, A., Alabi, C. A., Yen, Y., Heidel, J. D., & Ribas, A. (2010). Evidence of RNAi in humans from systemically administered siRNA via targeted nanoparticles. *Nature*, *464*(7291), 1067–1070. Available from https://doi.org/10.1038/nature08956.

Deng, Z. J., Liang, M., Monteiro, M., Toth, I., & Minchin, R. F. (2011). Nanoparticle-induced unfolding of fibrinogen promotes Mac-1 receptor activation and inflammation. *Nature Nanotechnology*, *6*(1), 39–44. Available from https://doi.org/10.1038/nnano.2010.250.

Dobrovolskaia, M. A., & McNeil, S. E. (2007). Immunological properties of engineered nanomaterials. *Nature Nanotechnology*, *2*(8), 469–478. Available from https://doi.org/10.1038/nnano.2007.223.

Dobrovolskaia, M. A., Aggarwal, P., Hall, J. B., & McNeil, S. E. (2008). Preclinical studies to understand nanoparticle interaction with the immune system and its potential effects on nanoparticle biodistribution. *Molecular Pharmaceutics*, *5*(4), 487–495. Available from https://doi.org/10.1021/mp800032f.

Dobrovolskaia, M. A., Germolec, D. R., & Weaver, J. L. (2009). Evaluation of nanoparticle immunotoxicity. *Nature Nanotechnology*, *4*(7), 411–414. Available from https://doi.org/10.1038/nnano.2009.175.

Dobrovolskaia, M. A., Neun, B. W., Clogston, J. D., Ding, H., Ljubimova, J., & McNeil, S. E. (2010). Ambiguities in applying traditional limulus amebocyte lysate tests to quantify endotoxin in nanoparticle formulations. *Nanomedicine*, *5*(4), 555–562. Available from https://doi.org/10.2217/nnm.10.29.

Doroud, D., Zahedifard, F., Vatanara, A., Najafabadi, A. R., & Rafati, S. (2011). Cysteine proteinase type I, encapsulated in solid lipid nanoparticles induces substantial protection against Leishmania major infection in C57BL/6 mice. *Parasite Immunology, 33*(6), 335–348. Available from https://doi.org/10.1111/j.1365-3024.2011.01289.x.

Dreaden, E. C., Mac key, M. A., Huang, X., Kang, B., & El-Sayed, M. A. (2011). Beating cancer in multiple ways using nanogold. *Chemical Society Reviews, 40*(7), 3391–3404. Available from https://doi.org/10.1039/c0cs00180e.

Dwivedi, P. D., Tripathi, A., Ansari, K. M., Shanker, R., & Das, M. (2011). Impact of nanoparticles on the immune system. *Journal of Biomedical Nanotechnology*, 7(1), 193–194. Available from https://doi.org/10.1166/jbn.2011.1264.

Elsabahy, M., & Wooley, K. L. (2012a). Design of polymeric nanoparticles for biomedical delivery applications. *Chemical Society Reviews, 41*(7), 2545–2561. Available from https://doi.org/10.1039/c2cs15327k.

Elsabahy, M., & Wooley, K. L. (2012b). Strategies toward well-defined polymer nanoparticles inspired by nature: Chemistry vs versatility. *Journal of Polymer Science, Part A: Polymer Chemistry, 50*(10), 1869–1880. Available from https://doi.org/10.1002/pola.25955.

Elsabahy, M., Dufresne, M.-H., & Leroux, J.-C. (2011). Polymeric micelles as versatile carriers for drugs and nucleic acids delivery. *Informa UK Limited*. Available from https://doi.org/10.1201/9780429111570-4.

Elsabahy, M., Wazen, N., Bayó-Puxan, N., Deleavey, G., Servant, M., Damha, M. J., & Leroux, J. C. (2009). Delivery of nucleic acids through the controlled disassembly of multifunctional nanocomplexes. *Advanced Functional Materials, 19*(24), 3862–3867. Available from https://doi.org/10.1002/adfm.200901139.

Elshal, M. F., & McCoy, J. P. (2006). Multiplex bead array assays: Performance evaluation and comparison of sensitivity to ELISA. *Methods, 38*(4), 317–323. Available from https://doi.org/10.1016/j.ymeth.2005.11.010.

Felber, A. E., Dufresne, M. H., & Leroux, J. C. (2012). PH-sensitive vesicles, polymeric micelles, and nanospheres prepared with polycarboxylates. *Advanced Drug Delivery Reviews, 64*(11), 979–992. Available from https://doi.org/10.1016/j.addr.2011.09.006.

Fifis, T., Gamvrellis, A., Crimeen-Irwin, B., Pietersz, G. A., Li, J., Mottram, P. L., McKenzie, I. F. C., & Plebanski, M. (2004). Size-dependent immunogenicity: Therapeutic and protective properties of nano-vaccines against tumors. *Journal of Immunology, 173*(5), 3148–3154. Available from https://doi.org/10.4049/jimmunol.173.5.3148.

Florindo, H. F., Pandit, S., Gonçalves, L. M. D., Alpar, H. O., & Almeida, A. J. (2009). New approach on the development of a mucosal vaccine against strangles: Systemic and mucosal immune responses in a mouse model. *Vaccine, 27*(8), 1230–1241. Available from https://doi.org/10.1016/j.vaccine.2008.12.004.

Freimark, B. D., Blezinger, H. P., Florack, V. J., Nordstrom, J. L., Long, S. D., Deshpande, D. S., Nochumson, S., & Petrak, K. L. (1998). Cationic lipids enhance cytokine and cell influx levels in the lung following administration of plasmid: Cationic lipid complexes. *Journal of Immunology, 160*(9), 4580–4586.

Fuhrmann, K., Schulz, J. D., Gauthier, M. A., & Leroux, J. C. (2012). PEG nanocages as non-sheddable stabilizers for drug nanocrystals. *ACS Nano, 6*(2), 1667–1676. Available from https://doi.org/10.1021/nn2046554.

Fukukawa, K. I., Rossin, R., Hagooly, A., Pressly, E. D., Hunt, J. N., Messmore, B. W., Wooley, K. L., Welch, M. J., & Hawker, C. J. (2008). Synthesis and characterization of core-shell star copolymers for in vivo PET imaging applications. *Biomacromolecules, 9*(4), 1329–1339. Available from https://doi.org/10.1021/bm7014152.

Gajewski, T. F., Pinnas, M., Wong, T., & Fitch, F. W. (1991). Murine Th1 and Th2 clones proliferate optimally in response to distinct antigen-presenting cell populations. *Journal of Immunology, 146*(6), 1750–1758.

Gaucher, G., Dufresne, M. H., Sant, V. P., Kang, N., Maysinger, D., & Leroux, J. C. (2005). Block copolymer micelles: Preparation, characterization and application in drug delivery. *Journal of Controlled Release, 109*(1–3), 169–188. Available from https://doi.org/10.1016/j.jconrel.2005.09.034.

Ghoneum, M., Ghoneum, A., & Gimzewski, J. (2010). Nanodiamond and nanoplatinum liquid, DPV576, activates human monocyte-derived dendritic cells in vitro. *Anticancer Research, 30*(10), 4075–4079.

Gianella, A., Jarzyna, P. A., Mani, V., Ramachandran, S., Calcagno, C., Tang, J., Kann, B., Dijk, W. J. R., Thijssen, V. L., Griffioen, A. W., Storm, G., Fayad, Z. A., & Mulder, W. J. M. (2011). Multifunctional nanoemulsion platform for imaging guided therapy evaluated in experimental cancer. *ACS Nano, 5*(6), 4422–4433. Available from https://doi.org/10.1021/nn103336a.

Gröne, A. (2002). Keratinocytes and cytokines. *Veterinary Immunology and Immunopathology, 88*(1–2), 1–12. Available from https://doi.org/10.1016/S0165-2427(02)00136-8.

Gui, S., Zhang, Z., Zheng, L., Cui, Y., Liu, X., Li, N., Sang, X., Sun, Q., Gao, G., Cheng, Z., Cheng, J., Wang, L., Tang, M., & Hong, F. (2011). Molecular mechanism of kidney injury of mice caused by exposure to titanium dioxide nanoparticles. *Journal of Hazardous Materials, 195*, 365–370. Available from https://doi.org/10.1016/j.jhazmat.2011.08.055.

Hamdy, S., Haddadi, A., Somayaji, V., Ruan, D., & Samuel, J. (2007). Pharmaceutical analysis of synthetic lipid A-based vaccine adjuvants in poly (d,l-lactic-co-glycolic acid) nanoparticle formulations. *Journal of Pharmaceutical and Biomedical Analysis, 44*(4), 914–923. Available from https://doi.org/10.1016/j.jpba.2007.03.010.

Hamdy, S., Molavi, O., Ma, Z., Haddadi, A., Alshamsan, A., Gobti, Z., Elhasi, S., Samuel, J., & Lavasanifar, A. (2008). Co-delivery of cancer-associated antigen and Toll-like receptor 4 ligand in PLGA nanoparticles induces potent CD8 + T cell-mediated anti-tumor immunity. *Vaccine, 26*(39), 5046–5057. Available from https://doi.org/10.1016/j.vaccine.2008.07.035.

Hamilton, R. F., Wu, N., Porter, D., Buford, M., Wolfarth, M., & Holian, A. (2009). Particle length-dependent titanium dioxide nanomaterials toxicity and bioactivity. *Particle and Fibre Toxicology, 6*. Available from https://doi.org/10.1186/1743-8977-6-35.

Hawkins, M. J., Soon-Shiong, P., & Desai, N. (2008). Protein nanoparticles as drug carriers in clinical medicine. *Advanced Drug Delivery Reviews, 60*(8), 876–885. Available from https://doi.org/10.1016/j.addr.2007.08.044.

Heng, B. C., Zhao, X., Tan, E. C., Khamis, N., Assodani, A., Xiong, S., Ruedl, C., Ng, K. W., & Loo, J. S. C. (2011). Evaluation of the cytotoxic and inflammatory potential of differentially shaped zinc oxide nanoparticles. *Archives of Toxicology, 85*(12), 1517–1528. Available from https://doi.org/10.1007/s00204-011-0722-1.

Huang, H. C., Barua, S., Sharma, G., Dey, S. K., & Rege, K. (2011). Inorganic nanoparticles for cancer imaging and therapy. *Journal of Controlled Release, 155*(3), 344–357. Available from https://doi.org/10.1016/j.jconrel.2011.06.004.

Hussain, S., Boland, S., Baeza-Squiban, A., Hamel, R., Thomassen, L. C. J., Martens, J. A., Billon-Galland, M. A., Fleury-Feith, J., Moisan, F., Pairon, J. C., & Marano, F. (2009). Oxidative stress and proinflammatory effects of carbon black and titanium dioxide nanoparticles: Role of particle surface area and internalized amount. *Toxicology, 260*(1–3), 142–149. Available from https://doi.org/10.1016/j.tox.2009.04.001.

Hussain, S., Vanoirbeek, J. A. J., & Hoet, P. H. M. (2012). Interactions of nanomaterials with the immune system. *WIREs Nanomedicine and Nanobiotechnology, 4*(2), 169–183. Available from https://doi.org/10.1002/wnan.166.

Hyde, S. C., Pringle, I. A., Abdullah, S., Lawton, A. E., Davies, L. A., Varathalingam, A., Nunez-Alonso, G., Green, A. M., Bazzani, R. P., Sumner-Jones, S. G., Chan, M., Li, H., Yew, N. S., Cheng, S. H., Christopher Boyd, A., Davies, J. C., Griesenbach, U.,

Porteous, D. J., Sheppard, D. N., ... Gill, D. R. (2008). CpG-free plasmids confer reduced inflammation and sustained pulmonary gene expression. *Nature Biotechnology*, *26*(5), 549−551. Available from https://doi.org/10.1038/nbt1399.

Iversen, T. G., Skotland, T., & Sandvig, K. (2011). Endocytosis and intracellular transport of nanoparticles: Present knowledge and need for future studies. *Nano Today*, *6*(2), 176−185. Available from https://doi.org/10.1016/j.nantod.2011.02.003.

Iwasaki, A., & Medzhitov, R. (2004). Toll-like receptor control of the adaptive immune responses. *Nature Immunology*, *5*(10), 987−995. Available from https://doi.org/10.1038/ni1112.

Javeed, A., Ashraf, M., Riaz, A., Ghafoor, A., Afzal, S., & Mukhtar, M. M. (2009). Paclitaxel and immune system. *European Journal of Pharmaceutical Sciences*, *38*(4), 283−290. Available from https://doi.org/10.1016/j.ejps.2009.08.009.

Jones, C. F., & Grainger, D. W. (2009). In vitro assessments of nanomaterial toxicity. *Advanced Drug Delivery Reviews*, *61*(6), 438−456. Available from https://doi.org/10.1016/j.addr.2009.03.005.

Judge, A., & MacLachlan, I. (2008). Overcoming the innate immune response to small interfering RNA. *Human Gene Therapy*, *19*(2), 111−124. Available from https://doi.org/10.1089/hum.2007.179.

Judge, A. D., Bola, G., Lee, A. C. H., & MacLachlan, I. (2006). Design of noninflammatory synthetic siRNA mediating potent gene silencing in vivo. *Molecular Therapy*, *13*(3), 494−505. Available from https://doi.org/10.1016/j.ymthe.2005.11.002.

Judge, A. D., Robbins, M., Tavakoli, I., Levi, J., Hu, L., Fronda, A., Ambegia, E., McClintock, K., & MacLachlan, I. (2009). Confirming the RNAi-mediated mechanism of action of siRNA-based cancer therapeutics in mice. *Journal of Clinical Investigation*, *119*(3), 661−673. Available from https://doi.org/10.1172/JCI37515.

Judge, A. D., Sood, V., Shaw, J. R., Fang, D., McClintock, K., & MacLachlan, I. (2005). Sequence-dependent stimulation of the mammalian innate immune response by synthetic siRNA. *Nature Biotechnology*, *23*(4), 457−462. Available from https://doi.org/10.1038/nbt1081.

Karikó, K., Bhuyan, P., Capodici, J., & Weissman, D. (2004). Small interfering RNAs mediate sequence-independent gene suppression and induce immune activation by signaling through toll-like receptor 3. *Journal of Immunology*, *172*(11), 6545−6549. Available from https://doi.org/10.4049/jimmunol.172.11.6545.

Kataoka, K., Harada, A., & Nagasaki, Y. (2001). Block copolymer micelles for drug delivery: Design, characterization and biological significance. *Advanced Drug Delivery Reviews*, *47*(1), 113−131. Available from https://doi.org/10.1016/S0169-409X(00)00124-1.

Kawai, T., & Akira, S. (2007). Signaling to NF-κB by Toll-like receptors. *Trends in Molecular Medicine*, *13*(11), 460−469. Available from https://doi.org/10.1016/j.molmed.2007.09.002.

Khan, I. H., Krishnan, V. V., Ziman, M., Janatpour, K., Wun, T., Luciv, P. A., & Tuscano, J. (2009). Comparison of multiplex suspension array large-panel kits for profiling cytokines and chemokines in rheumatoid arthritis patients. *Cytometry Part B - Clinical Cytometry*, *76*(3), 159−168. Available from https://doi.org/10.1002/cyto.b.20452.

Kidd, P. (2003). Th1/Th2 balance: The hypothesis, its limitations, and implications for health and disease. *Alternative Medicine Review*, *8*(3), 223−246.

Kim, B. H., Lee, Y. S., & Kang, K. S. (2003). The mechanism of retinol-induced irritation and its application to anti-irritant development. *Toxicology Letters*, *146*(1), 65−73. Available from https://doi.org/10.1016/j.toxlet.2003.09.001.

Kim, J. Y., Choung, S., Lee, E. J., Kim, Y. J., & Choi, Y. C. (2007). Immune activation by siRNA/liposome complexes in mice is sequence- independent: Lack of a role for toll-like receptor 3 signaling. *Molecules and Cells*, *24*(2), 247−254. Available from http://molcells.org/home/journal/include/downloadPdf.asp?articleuid = {C74B6235-4BC4-44D8-8424-6786EE61CBC3}.

Kim, T. H., Nah, J. W., Cho, M. H., Park, T. G., & Cho, N. S. (2006). Receptor-mediated gene delivery into antigen presenting cells using mannosylated chitosan/DNA nanoparticles. *Journal of Nanoscience and Nanotechnology*, *6*(9–10), 2796–2803. Available from https://doi.org/10.1166/jnn.2006.434.

Kocbach, A., Totlandsdal, A. I., Låg, M., Refsnes, M., & Schwarze, P. E. (2008). Differential binding of cytokines to environmentally relevant particles: A possible source for misinterpretation of in vitro results? *Toxicology Letters*, *176*(2), 131–137. Available from https://doi.org/10.1016/j.toxlet.2007.10.014.

Kokkonen, H., Söderström, I., Rocklöv, J., Hallmans, G., Lejon, K., & Dahlqvist, S. R. (2010). Up-regulation of cytokines and chemokines predates the onset of rheumatoid arthritis. *Arthritis and Rheumatism*, *62*(2), 383–391. Available from https://doi.org/10.1002/art.27186.

Kroll, A., Pillukat, M. H., Hahn, D., & Schnekenburger, J. (2009). Current in vitro methods in nanoparticle risk assessment: Limitations and challenges. *European Journal of Pharmaceutics and Biopharmaceutics*, *72*(2), 370–377. Available from https://doi.org/10.1016/j.ejpb.2008.08.009.

Kumar, M., Kong, X., Behera, A. K., Hellermann, G. R., Lockey, R. F., & Mohapatra, S. S. (2003). Chitosan IFN-gamma-pDNA nanoparticle (CIN) therapy for allergic asthma. *Genetic Vaccines and Therapy*, *1*.

Kutzler, M. A., & Weiner, D. B. (2008). DNA vaccines: Ready for prime time? *Nature Reviews Genetics*, *9*(10), 776–788. Available from https://doi.org/10.1038/nrg2432.

Lan, Q., Wang, S. S., Menashe, I., Armstrong, B., Zhang, Y., Hartge, P., Purdue, M. P., Holford, T. R., Morton, L. M., Kricker, A., Cerhan, J. R., Grulich, A., Cozen, W., Zahm, S. H., Yeager, M., Vajdic, C. M., Schenk, M., Leaderer, B., Yuenger, J., ... Rothman, N. (2011). Genetic variation in Th1/Th2 pathway genes and risk of non-Hodgkin lymphoma: A pooled analysis of three population-based case-control studies. *British Journal of Haematology*, *153*(3), 341–350. Available from https://doi.org/10.1111/j.1365-2141.2010.08424.x.

Lanier, L. (1991). In D.P., & A. I. Terr (Eds.), *Basic Human Immunology*. Appleton & Lange.

Larsen, S. T., Roursgaard, M., Jensen, K. A., & Nielsen, G. D. (2010). Nano titanium dioxide particles promote allergic sensitization and lung inflammation in mice. *Basic and Clinical Pharmacology and Toxicology*, *106*(2), 114–117. Available from https://doi.org/10.1111/j.1742-7843.2009.00473.x.

Lawrence, T. (2009). The nuclear factor NF-kappaB pathway in inflammation. *Cold Spring Harbor Perspectives Biology*, *1*.

Lee, J. H., Lee, K., Moon, S. H., Lee, Y., Park, T. G., & Cheon, J. (2009). All-in-one target-cell-specific magnetic nanoparticles for simultaneous molecular imaging and siRNA delivery. *Angewandte Chemie - International Edition*, *48*(23), 4174–4179. Available from https://doi.org/10.1002/anie.200805998.

Leng, S. X., McElhaney, J. E., Walston, J. D., Xie, D., Fedarko, N. S., & Kuchel, G. A. (2008). ELISA and multiplex technologies for cytokine measurement in inflammation and aging research. *Journals of Gerontology - Series A Biological Sciences and Medical Sciences*, *63*(8), 879–884. Available from https://doi.org/10.1093/gerona/63.8.879.

Li, C., & Wallace, S. (2008). Polymer-drug conjugates: Recent development in clinical oncology. *Advanced Drug Delivery Reviews*, *60*(8), 886–898. Available from https://doi.org/10.1016/j.addr.2007.11.009.

Li, J., Chen, Y. C., Tseng, Y. C., Mozumdar, S., & Huang, L. (2010). Biodegradable calcium phosphate nanoparticle with lipid coating for systemic siRNA delivery. *Journal of Controlled Release*, *142*(3), 416–421. Available from https://doi.org/10.1016/j.jconrel.2009.11.008.

Liu, T., Li, L., Fu, C., Liu, H., Chen, D., & Tang, F. (2012). Pathological mechanisms of liver injury caused by continuous intraperitoneal injection of silica nanoparticles. *Biomaterials*, *33*(7), 2399–2407. Available from https://doi.org/10.1016/j.biomaterials.2011.12.008.

Liu, Y., Jiao, F., Qiu, Y., Li, W., Lao, F., Zhou, G., Sun, B., Xing, G., Dong, J., Zhao, Y., Chai, Z., & Chen, C. (2009). The effect of Gd@C82(OH)22 nanoparticles on the release of Th1/Th2 cytokines and induction of TNF-α mediated cellular immunity. *Biomaterials, 30*(23–24), 3934–3945. Available from https://doi.org/10.1016/j.biomaterials.2009.04.001.

Liu, Z., Davis, C., Cai, W., He, L., Chen, X., & Dai, H. (2008). Circulation and long-term fate of functionalized, biocompatible single-walled carbon nanotubes in mice probed by Raman spectroscopy. *Proceedings of the National Academy of Sciences of the United States of America, 105* (5), 1410–1415. Available from https://doi.org/10.1073/pnas.0707654105.

Ma, C. S., Tangye, S. G., & Deenick, E. K. (2010). Human Th9 cells: Inflammatory cytokines modulate IL-9 production through the induction of IL-21. *Immunology and Cell Biology, 88*(6), 621–623. Available from https://doi.org/10.1038/icb.2010.73.

Mahvi, D. M., Henry, M. B., Albertini, M. R., Weber, S., Meredith, K., Schalch, H., Rakhmilevich, A., Hank, J., & Sondel, P. (2007). Intratumoral injection of IL-12 plasmid DNA - Results of a phase I/IB clinical trial. *Cancer Gene Therapy, 14*(8), 717–723. Available from https://doi.org/10.1038/sj.cgt.7701064.

Manolova, V., Flace, A., Bauer, M., Schwarz, K., Saudan, P., & Bachmann, M. F. (2008). Nanoparticles target distinct dendritic cell populations according to their size. *European Journal of Immunology, 38*(5), 1404–1413. Available from https://doi.org/10.1002/eji.200737984.

Marquis, B. J., Love, S. A., Braun, K. L., & Haynes, C. L. (2009). Analytical methods to assess nanoparticle toxicity. *Analyst, 134*(3), 425–439. Available from https://doi.org/10.1039/b818082b.

McNeil, S. E. (Ed.), (2011). *Characterization of nanoparticles intended for drug delivery*. New York: Human Press.

Medzhitov, R., Shevach, E. M., Trinchieri, G., Mellor, A. L., Munn, D. H., Gordon, S., Libby, P., Hansson, G. K., Shortman, K., Dong, C., Gabrilovich, D., Gabrysŏvá, L., Howes, A., & O'Garra, A. (2011). Highlights of 10 years of immunology in. *Nature Reviews Immunology. Nature Reviews Immunology, 11*(10), 693–702. Available from https://doi.org/10.1038/nri3063.

Meunier, E., Coste, A., Olagnier, D., Authier, H., Lefèvre, L., Dardenne, C., Bernad, J., Béraud, M., Flahaut, E., & Pipy, B. (2012). Double-walled carbon nanotubes trigger IL-1β release in human monocytes through Nlrp3 inflammasome activation. *Nanomedicine: Nanotechnology, Biology, and Medicine, 8*(6), 987–995. Available from https://doi.org/10.1016/j.nano.2011.11.004.

Minigo, G., Scholzen, A., Tang, C. K., Hanley, J. C., Kalkanidis, M., Pietersz, G. A., Apostolopoulos, V., & Plebanski, M. (2007). Poly-l-lysine-coated nanoparticles: A potent delivery system to enhance DNA vaccine efficacy. *Vaccine, 25*(7), 1316–1327. Available from https://doi.org/10.1016/j.vaccine.2006.09.086.

Moon, C., Park, H. J., Choi, Y. H., Park, E. M., Castranova, V., & Kang, J. L. (2010). Pulmonary inflammation after intraperitoneal administration of ultrafine titanium dioxide (TiO2) at rest or in lungs primed with lipopolysaccharide. *Journal of Toxicology and Environmental Health - Part A: Current Issues, 73*(5–6), 396–409. Available from https://doi.org/10.1080/15287390903486543.

Morand, E. F. (2007). Effects of glucocorticoids on inflammation and arthritis. *Current Opinion in Rheumatology, 19*(3), 302–307. Available from https://doi.org/10.1097/BOR.0b013e32805e87d0.

Morikawa, Y., Furotani, M., Matsuura, N., & Kakudo, K. (1993). The role of antigen-presenting cells in the regulation of delayed-type hypersensitivity: II. Epidermal langerhans' cells and peritoneal exudate macrophages. *Cellular Immunology, 152*(1), 200–210. Available from https://doi.org/10.1006/cimm.1993.1279.

Morishige, T., Yoshioka, Y., Inakura, H., Tanabe, A., Narimatsu, S., Yao, X., Monobe, Y., Imazawa, T., Tsunoda, S. I., Tsutsumi, Y., Mukai, Y., Okada, N., & Nakagawa,

S. (2012). Suppression of nanosilica particle-induced inflammation by surface modification of the particles. *Archives of Toxicology*, *86*(8), 1297–1307. Available from https://doi.org/10.1007/s00204-012-0823-5.

Morrissey, D. V., Lockridge, J. A., Shaw, L., Blanchard, K., Jensen, K., Breen, W., Hartsough, K., Machemer, L., Radka, S., Jadhav, V., Vaish, N., Zinnen, S., Vargeese, C., Bowman, K., Shaffer, C. S., Jeffs, L. B., Judge, A., MacLachlan, I., & Polisky, B. (2005). Potent and persistent in vivo anti-HBV activity of chemically modified siRNAs. *Nature Biotechnology*, *23*(8), 1002–1007. Available from https://doi.org/10.1038/nbt1122.

Mosmann, T. R., Cherwinski, H., Bond, M. W., Giedlin, M. A., & Coffman, R. L. (1986). Two types of murine helper T cell clone. I. Definition according to profiles of lymphokine activities and secreted proteins. *Journal of Immunology*, *175*, 5–14.

Mottram, P. L., Leong, D., Crimeen-Irwin, B., Gloster, S., Xiang, S. D., Meanger, J., Ghildyal, R., Vardaxis, N., & Plebanski, M. (2007). Type 1 and 2 immunity following vaccination is influenced by nanoparticle size: Formulation of a model vaccine for respiratory syncytial virus. *Molecular Pharmaceutics*, *4*(1), 73–84. Available from https://doi.org/10.1021/mp060096p.

Movassaghian, S., Moghimi, H. R., Shirazi, F. H., & Torchilin, V. P. (2011). Dendrosome-dendriplex inside liposomes: As a gene delivery system. *Journal of Drug Targeting*, *19*(10), 925–932. Available from https://doi.org/10.3109/1061186X.2011.628396.

Moynagh, P. N. (2003). Toll-like receptor signalling pathways as key targets for mediating the anti-inflammatory and immunosuppressive effects of glucocorticoids. *Journal of Endocrinology*, *179*(2), 139–144. Available from https://doi.org/10.1677/joe.0.1790139.

Munoz, C., Misset, B., Fitting, C., Blériot, J. P., Carlet, J., & Cavaillon, J. M. (1991). Dissociation between plasma and monocyte-associated cytokines during sepsis. *European Journal of Immunology*, *21*(9), 2177–2184. Available from https://doi.org/10.1002/eji.1830210928.

Murray, A. R., Kisin, E., Inman, A., Young, S. H., Muhammed, M., Burks, T., Uheida, A., Tkach, A., Waltz, M., Castranova, V., Fadeel, B., Kagan, V. E., Riviere, J. E., Monteiro-Riviere, N., & Shvedova, A. A. (2013). Oxidative stress and dermal toxicity of iron oxide nanoparticles in vitro. *Cell Biochemistry and Biophysics*. Available from https://doi.org/10.1007/s12013-12012-19367-12019.

Murray, A. R., Kisin, E., Leonard, S. S., Young, S. H., Kommineni, C., Kagan, V. E., Castranova, V., & Shvedova, A. A. (2009). Oxidative stress and inflammatory response in dermal toxicity of single-walled carbon nanotubes. *Toxicology*, *257*(3), 161–171. Available from https://doi.org/10.1016/j.tox.2008.12.023.

Nazmi, A., Dutta, K., Basu, A., & Singh, S. K. (2010). Antiviral and neuroprotective role of octaguanidinium dendrimer-conjugated morpholino oligomers in Japanese encephalitis. *PLoS Neglected Tropical Diseases*, *4*(11), e892. Available from https://doi.org/10.1371/journal.pntd.0000892.

Neurath, M. F., Finotto, S., & Glimcher, L. H. (2002). The role of TH1/TH2 polarization in mucosal immunity. *Nature Medicine*, *8*(6), 567–573. Available from https://doi.org/10.1038/nm0602-567.

Nguyen, T. H. T., & Casale, T. B. (2011). Immune modulation for treatment of allergic disease. *Immunological Reviews*, *242*(1), 258–271. Available from https://doi.org/10.1111/j.1600-065X.2011.01034.x.

Nishiyama, N., & Kataoka, K. (2006). Current state, achievements, and future prospects of polymeric micelles as nanocarriers for drug and gene delivery. *Pharmacology and Therapeutics*, *112*(3), 630–648. Available from https://doi.org/10.1016/j.pharmthera.2006.05.006.

Nyström, A. M., & Wooley, K. L. (2011). The importance of chemistry in creating well-defined nanoscopic embedded therapeutics: Devices capable of the dual functions of imaging and therapy. *Accounts of Chemical Research*, *44*(10), 969–978. Available from https://doi.org/10.1021/ar200097k.

Pasare, C., & Medzhitov, R. (2005). *Toll-like receptors: Linking innate and adaptive immunity, Advances in Experimental Medicine and Biology* (Vol. 560, pp. 11–18). Springer Science and Business Media Deutschland GmbH. Available from https://doi.org/10.1007/0-387-24180-9_2.

Powers, M. R., Davies, M. H., & Eubanks, J. P. (2005). Increased expression of chemokine KC, an interleukin-8 homologue, in a model of oxygen-induced retinopathy. *Current Eye Research, 30*(4), 299–307. Available from https://doi.org/10.1080/02713680590923276.

Prato, M., Kostarelos, K., & Bianco, A. (2008). Functionalized carbon nanotubes in drug design and discovery. *Accounts of Chemical Research, 41*(1), 60–68. Available from https://doi.org/10.1021/ar700089b.

Pressly, E. D., Rossin, R., Hagooly, A., Fukukawa, K. I., Messmore, B. W., Welch, M. J., Wooley, K. L., Lamm, M. S., Hule, R. A., Pochan, D. J., & Hawker, C. J. (2007). Structural effects on the biodistribution and positron emission tomograpgy (PET) imaging of well-defined 64Cu-labeled nanoparticles comprised of amphiphilic block graft copolymers. *Biomacromolecules, 8*(10), 3126–3134. Available from https://doi.org/10.1021/bm700541e.

Pulskamp, K., Diabate, S., & Krug, H. (2007). Carbon nanotubes show no sign of acute toxicity but induce intracellular reactive oxygen species in dependence on contaminants. *Toxicology Letters, 168*(1), 58–74. Available from https://doi.org/10.1016/j.toxlet.2006.11.001.

Rajananthanan, P., Attard, G. S., Sheikh, N. A., & Morrow, W. J. W. (1999). Novel aggregate structure adjuvants modulate lymphocyte proliferation and Th1 and Th2 cytokine profiles in ovalbumin immunized mice. *Vaccine, 18*(1–2), 140–152. Available from https://doi.org/10.1016/S0264-410X(99)00213-3.

Reddy, S. T., Van Der Vlies, A. J., Simeoni, E., Angeli, V., Randolph, G. J., O'Neil, C. P., Lee, L. K., Swartz, M. A., & Hubbell, J. A. (2007). Exploiting lymphatic transport and complement activation in nanoparticle vaccines. *Nature Biotechnology, 25*(10), 1159–1164. Available from https://doi.org/10.1038/nbt1332.

Reisetter, A. C., Stebounova, L. V., Baltrusaitis, J., Powers, L., Gupta, A., Grassian, V. H., & Monick, M. M. (2011). Induction of inflammasome-dependent pyroptosis by carbon black nanoparticles. *Journal of Biological Chemistry, 286*(24), 21844–21852. Available from https://doi.org/10.1074/jbc.M111.238519.

Rettig, L., Haen, S. P., Bittermann, A. G., Von Boehmer, L., Curioni, A., Krämer, S. D., Knuth, A., & Pascolo, S. (2010). Particle size and activation threshold: A new dimension of danger signaling. *Blood, 115*(22), 4533–4541. Available from https://doi.org/10.1182/blood-2009-11-247817.

Rottembourg, D., Filippi, C. M., Bresson, D., Ehrhardt, K., Estes, E. A., Oldham, J. E., & Von Herrath, M. G. (2010). Essential role for TLR9 in prime but not prime-boost plasmid DNA vaccination to activate dendritic cells and protect from lethal viral infection. *Journal of Immunology, 184*(12), 7100–7107. Available from https://doi.org/10.4049/jimmunol.0803935.

Ruiz, F. E., Clancy, J. P., Perricone, M. A., Bebok, Z., Hong, J. S., Cheng, S. H., Meeker, D. P., Young, K. R., Schoumacher, R. A., Weatherly, M. R., Wing, L., Morris, J. E., Sindel, L., Rosenberg, M., Van Ginkel, F. W., McGhee, J. R., Kelly, D., Lyrene, R. K., & Sorscher, E. J. (2001). A clinical inflammatory syndrome attributable to aerosolized lipid-DNA administration in cystic fibrosis. *Human Gene Therapy, 12*(7), 751–761. Available from https://doi.org/10.1089/104303401750148667.

Ryman-Rasmussen, J. P., Riviere, J. E., & Monteiro-Riviere, N. A. (2007). Surface coatings determine cytotoxicity and irritation potential of quantum dot nanoparticles in epidermal keratinocytes. *Journal of Investigative Dermatology, 127*(1), 143–153. Available from https://doi.org/10.1038/sj.jid.5700508.

Sandberg, W. J., Låg, M., Holme, J. A., Friede, B., Gualtieri, M., Kruszewski, M., Schwarze, P. E., Skuland, T., & Refsnes, M. (2012). Comparison of non-crystalline silica nanoparticles in IL-1β release from macrophages. *Particle and Fibre Toxicology, 9*. Available from https://doi.org/10.1186/1743-8977-9-32.

Schanen, B. C., Karakoti, A. S., Seal, S., Drake, D. R., Warren, W. L., & Self, W. T. (2009). Exposure to titanium dioxide nanomaterials provokes inflammation of an in vitro human immune construct. *ACS Nano, 3*(9), 2523–2532. Available from https://doi.org/10.1021/nn900403h.

Scheule, R. K., St. George, J. A., Bagley, R. G., Marshall, J., Kaplan, J. M., Akita, G. Y., Wang, K. X., Lee, E. R., Harris, D. J., Jiang, C., Yew, N. S., Smith, A. E., & Cheng, S. H. (1997). Basis of pulmonary toxicity associated with cationic lipid-mediated gene transfer to the mammalian lung. *Human Gene Therapy, 8*(6), 689–707. Available from https://doi.org/10.1089/hum.1997.8.6-689.

Schneider, C. K., Kalinke, U., & Löwer, J. (2006). TGN1412 - A regulator's perspective [1]. *Nature Biotechnology, 24*(5), 493–496. Available from https://doi.org/10.1038/nbt0506-493.

Semple, S. C., Akinc, A., Chen, J., Sandhu, A. P., Mui, B. L., Cho, C. K., Sah, D. W. Y., Stebbing, D., Crosley, E. J., Yaworski, E., Hafez, I. M., Dorkin, J. R., Qin, J., Lam, K., Rajeev, K. G., Wong, K. F., Jeffs, L. B., Nechev, L., Eisenhardt, M. L., ... Hope, M. J. (2010). Rational design of cationic lipids for siRNA delivery. *Nature Biotechnology, 28*(2), 172–176. Available from https://doi.org/10.1038/nbt.1602.

Sepp-Lorenzino, L., & Ruddy, M. K. (2008). Challenges and opportunities for local and systemic delivery of siRNA and antisense oligonucleotides. *Clinical Pharmacology and Therapeutics, 84*(5), 628–632. Available from https://doi.org/10.1038/clpt.2008.174.

Shi, J., Xiao, Z., Kamaly, N., & Farokhzad, O. C. (2011). Self-assembled targeted nanoparticles: Evolution of technologies and bench to bedside translation. *Accounts of Chemical Research, 44*(10), 1123–1134. Available from https://doi.org/10.1021/ar200054n.

Shin, J. A., Lee, E. J., Seo, S. M., Kim, H. S., Kang, J. L., & Park, E. M. (2010). Nanosized titanium dioxide enhanced inflammatory responses in the septic brain of mouse. *Neuroscience, 165*(2), 445–454. Available from https://doi.org/10.1016/j.neuroscience.2009.10.057.

Shiraki, T., Takayama, E., Magari, H., Nakata, T., Maekita, T., Enomoto, S., Mori, Y., Shingaki, N., Moribata, K., Deguchi, H., Ueda, K., Inoue, I., Mizuno-Kamiya, M., Yashiro, K., Iguchi, M., Tamai, H., Kameyama, Y., Kato, J., Kondoh, N., & Ichinose, M. (2011). Altered cytokine levels and increased CD4 + CD57 + T cells in the peripheral blood of hepatitis C virus-related hepatocellular carcinoma patients. *Oncology Reports, 26*(1), 201–208. Available from https://doi.org/10.3892/or.2011.1258.

Shvedova, A. A., Kisin, E. R., Mercer, R., Murray, A. R., Johnson, V. J., Potapovich, A. I., Tyurina, Y. Y., Gorelik, O., Arepalli, S., Schwegler-Berry, D., Hubbs, A. F., Antonini, J., Evans, D. E., Ku, B. K., Ramsey, D., Maynard, A., Kagan, V. E., Castranova, V., & Baron, P. (2005). Unusual inflammatory and fibrogenic pulmonary responses to single-walled carbon nanotubes in mice. *American Journal of Physiology – Lung Cellular and Molecular Physiology, 289*(5), L698–L708. Available from https://doi.org/10.1152/ajplung.00084.2005.

Simard, P., & Leroux, J.-C. (2010). In vivo evaluation of pH-sensitive polymer-based immunoliposomes targeting the CD33 antigen. *Molecular Pharmaceutics*, 1098–1107. Available from https://doi.org/10.1021/mp900261m.

Singer, J. W. (2005). Paclitaxel poliglumex (XYOTAXTM, CT-2103): A macromolecular taxane. *Journal of Controlled Release, 109*(1–3), 120–126. Available from https://doi.org/10.1016/j.jconrel.2005.09.033.

Singer, J. W., Shaffer, S., Baker, B., Bernareggi, A., Stromatt, S., Nienstedt, D., & Besman, M. (2005). Paclitaxel poliglumex (XYOTAX; CT-2103): An intracellularly targeted taxane. *Anti-Cancer Drugs, 16*(3), 243–254. Available from https://doi.org/10.1097/00001813-200503000-00003.

Singh, J., Pandit, S., Bramwell, V. W., & Alpar, H. O. (2006). Diphtheria toxoid loaded poly-(ε-caprolactone) nanoparticles as mucosal vaccine delivery systems. *Methods, 38* (2), 96–105. Available from https://doi.org/10.1016/j.ymeth.2005.11.003.

Sood, A., Salih, S., Roh, D., Lacharme-Lora, L., Parry, M., Hardiman, B., Keehan, R., Grummer, R., Winterhager, E., Gokhale, P. J., Andrews, P. W., Abbott, C., Forbes, K., Westwood, M., Aplin, J. D., Ingham, E., Papageorgiou, I., Berry, M., Liu, J., ... Case, C. P. (2011). Signalling of DNA damage and cytokines across cell barriers exposed to nanoparticles depends on barrier thickness. *Nature Nanotechnology, 6*(12), 824–833. Available from https://doi.org/10.1038/nnano.2011.188.

Stanberry, L. R., Simon, J. K., Johnson, C., Robinson, P. L., Morry, J., Flack, M. R., Gracon, S., Myc, A., Hamouda, T., & Baker, J. R. (2012). Safety and immunogenicity of a novel nanoemulsion mucosal adjuvant W 805EC combined with approved seasonal influenza antigens. *Vaccine, 30*(2), 307–316. Available from https://doi.org/10.1016/j.vaccine.2011.10.094.

Stebbings, R., Findlay, L., Edwards, C., Eastwood, D., Bird, C., North, D., Mistry, Y., Dilger, P., Liefooghe, E., Cludts, I., Fox, B., Tarrant, G., Robinson, J., Meager, T., Dolman, C., Thorpe, S. J., Bristow, A., Wadhwa, M., Thorpe, R., & Poole, S. (2007). \Cytokine storm\ in the Phase I trial of monoclonal antibody TGN1412: Better understanding the causes to improve preclinical testing of immunotherapeutics. *Journal of Immunology, 179*(5), 3325–3331. Available from https://doi.org/10.4049/jimmunol.179.5.3325.

Stone, V., Johnston, H., & Schins, R. P. F. (2009). Development of in vitro systems for nanotoxicology: Methodological considerations. *Critical Reviews in Toxicology, 39*(7), 613–626. Available from https://doi.org/10.1080/10408440903120975.

Sun, B., Wang, X., Ji, Z., Li, R., & Xia, T. (2013). NLRP3 inflammasome activation induced by engineered nanomaterials. *Small, 9*(9–10), 1595–1607. Available from https://doi.org/10.1002/smll.201201962.

Sun, G., Hagooly, A., Xu, J., Nystrom, A. M., Li, Z., Rossin, R., Moore, D. A., Wooley, K. L., & Welch, M. J. (1997). Facile, efficient approach to accomplish tunable chemistries and variable biodistributions for shell cross-linked nanoparticles. *Biomacromolecules, 9*.

Suntharalingam, G., Perry, M. R., Ward, S., Brett, S. J., Castello-Cortes, A., Brunner, M. D., & Panoskaltsis, N. (2006). Cytokine storm in a phase 1 trial of the anti-CD28 monoclonal antibody TGN1412. *New England Journal of Medicine, 355*(10), 1018–1028. Available from https://doi.org/10.1056/NEJMoa063842.

Tacken, P. J., Zeelenberg, I. S., Cruz, L. J., Van Hout-Kuijer, M. A., Van De Glind, G., Fokkink, R. G., Lambeck, A. J. A., & Figdor, C. G. (2011). Targeted delivery of TLR ligands to human and mouse dendritic cells strongly enhances adjuvanticity. *Blood, 118*(26), 6836–6844. Available from https://doi.org/10.1182/blood-2011-07-367615.

Takeda, K., Kaisho, T., & Akira, S. (2003). Toll-like receptors. *Annual Review of Immunology, 21*, 335–376. Available from https://doi.org/10.1146/annurev.immunol.21.120601.141126.

Tan, Y., Li, S., Pitt, B. R., & Huang, L. (1999). The inhibitory role of CpG immunostimulatory motifs in cationic lipid vector-mediated transgene expression in vivo. *Human Gene Therapy, 10*(13), 2153–2161. Available from https://doi.org/10.1089/10430349950017149.

Tao, W., Mao, X., Davide, J. P., Ng, B., Cai, M., Burke, P. A., Sachs, A. B., & Sepp-Lorenzino, L. (2011). Mechanistically probing lipid-sirna nanoparticle-associated toxicities identifies jak inhibitors effective in mitigating multifaceted toxic responses. *Molecular Therapy, 19*(3), 567–575. Available from https://doi.org/10.1038/mt.2010.282.

Tashiro, H., Shimokawa, H., Yamamoto, K., Momohara, M., Tada, H., & Takeshita, A. (1997). Altered plasma levels of cytokines in patients with ischemic heart disease. *Coronary Artery Disease, 8*(3–4), 143–147. Available from https://doi.org/10.1097/00019501-199703000-00004.

Thasneem, Y. M., Sajeesh, S., & Sharma, C. P. (2011). Effect of thiol functionalization on the hemo-compatibility of PLGA nanoparticles. *Journal of Biomedical Materials Research - Part A*, *99*(4), 607−617. Available from https://doi.org/10.1002/jbm.a.33220.

Thomas, C., Rawat, A., Hope-Weeks, L., & Ahsan, F. (2011). Aerosolized PLA and PLGA nanoparticles enhance humoral, mucosal and cytokine responses to hepatitis B vaccine. *Molecular Pharmaceutics*, *8*(2), 405−415. Available from https://doi.org/10.1021/mp100255c.

Torchilin, V. P. (2007). Micellar nanocarriers: Pharmaceutical perspectives. *Pharmaceutical Research*, *24*(1), 1−16. Available from https://doi.org/10.1007/s11095-006-9132-0.

Tsao, N., Kanakamma, P. P., Luh, T. Y., Chou, C. K., & Lei, H. Y. (1999). Inhibition of Escherichia coli-induced meningitis by carboxyfullerence. *Antimicrobial Agents and Chemotherapy*, *43*(9), 2273−2277. Available from https://doi.org/10.1128/aac.43.9.2273.

Val, S., Hussain, S., Boland, S., Hamel, R., Baeza-Squiban, A., & Marano, F. (2009). Carbon black and titanium dioxide nanoparticles induce pro-inflammatory responses in bronchial epithelial cells: Need for multiparametric evaluation due to adsorption artifacts. *Inhalation Toxicology*, *21*(1), 115−122. Available from https://doi.org/10.1080/08958370902942533.

Vallhov, H., Qin, J., Johansson, S. M., Ahlborg, N., Muhammed, M. A., Scheynius, A., & Gabrielsson, S. (2006). The importance of an endotoxin-free environment during the production of nanoparticles used in medical applications. *Nano Letters*, *6*(8), 1682−1686. Available from https://doi.org/10.1021/nl060860z.

Veranth, J. M., Kaser, E. G., Veranth, M. M., Koch, M., & Yost, G. S. (2007). Cytokine responses of human lung cells (BEAS-2B) treated with micron-sized and nanoparticles of metal oxides compared to soil dusts. *Particle and Fibre Toxicology*, *4*. Available from https://doi.org/10.1186/1743-8977-4-2.

Vistnes, M., Wæhre, A., Nygård, S., Sjaastad, I., Andersson, K. B., Husberg, C., & Christensen, G. (2010). Circulating cytokine levels in mice with heart failure are etiology dependent. *Journal of Applied Physiology*, *108*(5), 1357−1364. Available from https://doi.org/10.1152/japplphysiol.01084.2009.

Von Maltzahn, G., Park, J. H., Lin, K. Y., Singh, N., Schwöppe, C., Mesters, R., Berdel, W. E., Ruoslahti, E., Sailor, M. J., & Bhatia, S. N. (2011). Nanoparticles that communicate in vivo to amplify tumour targeting. *Nature Materials*, *10*(7), 545−552. Available from https://doi.org/10.1038/nmat3049.

Waes. (2007). Nuclear factor-kappaB in development, prevention, and therapy of cancer. *Clinical Cancer Research*, *13*, 1076−1082.

Wang, J., Chen, B., Jin, N., Xia, G., Chen, Y., Zhou, Y., Cai, X., Ding, J., Li, X., & Wang, X. (2011). The changes of T lymphocytes and cytokines in ICR mice fed with Fe3O4 magnetic nanoparticles. *International Journal of Nanomedicine*, *6*, 605−610.

Watts, J. K., Deleavey, G. F., & Damha, M. J. (2008). Chemically modified siRNA: Tools and applications. *Drug Discovery Today*, *13*(19−20), 842−855. Available from https://doi.org/10.1016/j.drudis.2008.05.007.

Witzmann, F. A., & Monteiro-Riviere, N. A. (2006). Multi-walled carbon nanotube exposure alters protein expression in human keratinocytes. *Nanomedicine: Nanotechnology, Biology, and Medicine*, *2*(3), 158−168. Available from https://doi.org/10.1016/j.nano.2006.07.005.

Wolff, J. A., & Rozema, D. B. (2008). Breaking the bonds: Non-viral vectors become chemically dynamic. *Molecular Therapy*, *16*(1), 8−15. Available from https://doi.org/10.1038/sj.mt.6300326.

Wolfrum, C., Shi, S., Jayaprakash, K. N., Jayaraman, M., Wang, G., Pandey, R. K., Rajeev, K. G., Nakayama, T., Charrise, K., Ndungo, E. M., Zimmermann, T., Koteliansky, V., Manoharan, M., & Stoffel, M. (2007). Mechanisms and optimization of in vivo delivery of lipophilic siRNAs. *Nature Biotechnology*, *25*(10), 1149−1157. Available from https://doi.org/10.1038/nbt1339.

Yang, E. J., Kim, S., Kim, J. S., & Choi, I. H. (2012). Inflammasome formation and IL-1β release by human blood monocytes in response to silver nanoparticles. *Biomaterials*, *33* (28), 6858–6867. Available from https://doi.org/10.1016/j.biomaterials.2012.06.016.

Yeung, T. K., Germond, C., Chen, X., & Wang, Z. (1999). The mode of action of Taxol: Apoptosis at low concentration and necrosis at high concentration. *Biochemical and Biophysical Research Communications*, *263*(2), 398–404. Available from https://doi.org/10.1006/bbrc.1999.1375.

Yew, N. S., Wang, K. X., Przybylska, M., Bagley, R. G., Stedman, M., Marshall, J., Scheule, R. K., & Cheng, S. H. (1999). Contribution of plasmid DNA to inflammation in the lung after administration of cationic lipid:pDNA complexes. *Human Gene Therapy*, *10*(2), 223–234. Available from https://doi.org/10.1089/10430349950019011.

Yoo, J. W., Irvine, D. J., Discher, D. E., & Mitragotri, S. (2011). Bio-inspired, bioengineered and biomimetic drug delivery carriers. *Nature Reviews Drug Discovery*, *10*(7), 521–535. Available from https://doi.org/10.1038/nrd3499.

Yoshida, H., Nishikawa, M., Yasuda, S., Mizuno, Y., Toyota, H., Kiyota, T., Takahashi, R., & Takakura, Y. (2009). TLR9-dependent systemic interferon-β production by intravenous injection of plasmid DNA/cationic liposome complex in mice. *Journal of Gene Medicine*, *11*(8), 708–717. Available from https://doi.org/10.1002/jgm.1348.

Zhang, K., Fang, H., Shen, G., Taylor, J. S. A., & Wooley, K. L. (2009). Well-defined cationic shell crosslinked nanoparticles for efficient delivery of DNA or peptide nucleic acids. *Proceedings of the American Thoracic Society*, *6*(5), 450–457. Available from https://doi.org/10.1513/pats.200902-010AW.

Zhang, K., Fang, H., Wang, Z., Li, Z., Taylor, J. S. A., & Wooley, K. L. (2010). Structure-activity relationships of cationic shell-crosslinked knedel-like nanoparticles: Shell composition and transfection efficiency/cytotoxicity. *Biomaterials*, *31*(7), 1805–1813. Available from https://doi.org/10.1016/j.biomaterials.2009.10.033.

Zhang, L. W., Yu, W. W., Colvin, V. L., & Monteiro-Riviere, N. A. (2008). Biological interactions of quantum dot nanoparticles in skin and in human epidermal keratinocytes. *Toxicology and Applied Pharmacology*, *228*(2), 200–211. Available from https://doi.org/10.1016/j.taap.2007.12.022.

Zimmermann, T. S., Lee, A. C. H., Akinc, A., Bramlage, B., Bumcrot, D., Fedoruk, M. N., Harborth, J., Heyes, J. A., Jeffs, L. B., John, M., Judge, A. D., Lam, K., McClintock, K., Nechev, L. V., Palmer, L. R., Racie, T., Röhl, I., Seiffert, S., Shanmugam, S., ... MacLachlan, I. (2006). RNAi-mediated gene silencing in non-human primates. *Nature*, *441*(1), 111–114. Available from https://doi.org/10.1038/nature04688.

Zitvogel, L., Apetoh, L., Ghiringhelli, F., & Kroemer, G. (2008). Immunological aspects of cancer chemotherapy. *Nature Reviews Immunology*, *8*(1), 59–73. Available from https://doi.org/10.1038/nri2216.

Zolnik, B. S., González-Fernández, A., Sadrieh, N., & Dobrovolskaia, M. A. (2010). Minireview: Nanoparticles and the immune system. *Endocrinology*, *151*(2), 458–465. Available from https://doi.org/10.1210/en.2009-1082.

CHAPTER 4

Methods for evaluation of the immunomodulatory effects of nanoparticles*

Mahmoud Elsabahy[1,2,3] and Karen L. Wooley[2]
[1]School of Biotechnology and Science Academy, Badr University in Cairo, Badr City, Cairo, Egypt
[2]Department of Chemistry, Laboratory for Synthetic-Biologic Interactions, Texas A&M University, College Station, TX, United States
[3]Misr University for Science and Technology, 6th of October City, Giza, Egypt

4.1 Introduction

Nanoparticles have widespread pharmaceutical and clinical applications, where safety and interactions with biomolecules are of critical significance (Elsabahy et al., 2015; Mitragotri et al., 2017; Mohamed et al., 2017). The type and composition of nanomaterials play a pivotal role in modulating the immune system, which may compromise therapeutic outcomes and can be life-threatening, in particular, when the immunomodulation is unintentional (Elsabahy & Wooley, 2013, 2015). Advances in multiplexing techniques and polychromatic flow cytometry have enabled the profiling of several hundreds of biomarkers in a few microliter sample volumes, with several existing limitations (Jani et al., 2016). Multiplexing assays for evaluating the immunotoxicity of these biomaterials are usually performed using the same approach utilized for small molecules. However, there are key differences in the physicochemical and biological characteristics between small molecules and large/assembled structures, which should not be overlooked (Elsabahy & Wooley, 2018; Elsabahy et al., 2013). In particular, the ability of assembled structures and particles to adsorb biomarkers on their surfaces and/or sequester them into their internal domains, in contrast to small molecules, is one of the main obstacles that may influence the accuracy of the multiplexing strategies for

* Adapted with permission from Elsabahy, M., Wooley, K. L., Hendricksen, A. & Oh, K. (2019). Multiplexing techniques for measurement of the immunomodulatory effects of particulate materials: Precautions when testing micro- and nano-particles. Methods, 158, 81-85. https://doi.org/10.1016/j.ymeth.2019.01.006.

Immunomodulatory Effects of Nanomaterials
DOI: https://doi.org/10.1016/B978-0-323-90604-3.00004-8

quantitative assessment of the expression of biomarkers after treatment with particulate materials. We have recently reported on the necessity for a reassessment of immunotoxicity of nanomaterials, and some important precautions to account for the differences in behavior between assembled/macromolecular structures and small molecules (Elsabahy & Wooley, 2018). The experimental details and precautions described herein can allow for precise evaluation of biomarker expression in response to particulate materials, pharmaceuticals, and medical devices and should be taken into careful consideration in preclinical and clinical studies and other processes that involve the use of multiplexing techniques.

4.2 Multiplexing technique for evaluation of particulate materials

There are several strategies that can be utilized for the evaluation of biomarkers in response to treatment with various biological agents. For instance, aggregation-induced emission-active functional materials have been extensively used for fluorescence sensing and biological imaging and thus could be utilized as fluorescence signals for biomarkers detection (Mao et al., 2019; Shi et al., 2017; Zhang et al., 2014). However, a focus is being given here on the use of the multiplexing technique as an efficient and commonly exploited strategy for the simultaneous detection of hundreds of biomarkers for the biological assessment of particulate materials. This article does not include the details of biological sample preparation, but rather the experimental methods and considerations during the analysis and quantification of expressed biomarkers in biological samples after in vitro or in vivo treatment with the tested biomaterials [summary of the procedures is illustrated in Fig. 4.1 (Elsabahy & Wooley, 2013)]. Prior training on pipetting is necessary for nonskilled personnel because these experiments are extremely sensitive to accurate volumes. Vortexing is an important step for several of the assay components before their use, particularly, for the magnetic beads. Selection of the controls is also critical for accurate data interpretation. Controls could be supernatants from cells treated with phosphate-buffered saline (PBS) or serum/plasma from animals injected with PBS. For comparison with other sets of materials (from the same or different laboratories), concentration of the tested materials, incubation time, or blood withdrawal time, together with other conditions, should be comparable.

Endotoxin contents should be measured before treatment of cells or animals with the tested materials. Presence of endotoxin in the samples may induce the release of several cytokines and, thus result in biased data. To

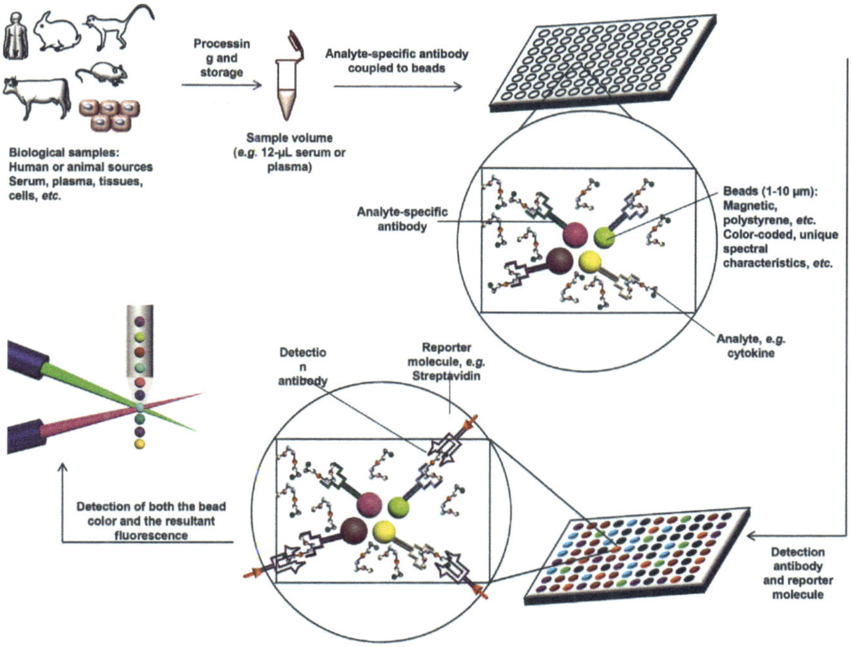

Figure 4.1 Schematic representation of the steps of multiplex assay for the simultaneous detection and measurements of biomarkers in biological samples of various sources. Detailed procedures are not included in this schematic diagram and the detection methods (e.g., color code vs fluorescence, or the use of various reporters, or the flow cytometric detection) vary depending on the specific instrument and kit utilized for the assay. *Reproduced by permission of the Royal Society of Chemistry (Elsabahy, M., & Wooley, K.L. (2013). Cytokines as biomarkers of nanoparticle immunotoxicity. Chemical Society Reviews, 42(12), 5552–5576. https://doi.org/10.1039/c3cs60064e).*

BOX 4.1 Minimizing contamination of the tested materials with endotoxins

Use endotoxin-free water, pipettes, tubes, etc.

Sterilize materials as much as possible.

Work under biological safety cabinets.

Seal or cover dialysis and stirring containers (by use of, e.g., parafilm, aluminum foils, etc.).

minimize the presence of endotoxins in the samples, clean procedures shall be used throughout the sample preparation process. Useful hints are provided to minimize the contamination of samples with endotoxins (Box 4.1).

The initial experiment described herein is designed to be carried out in a 96-well plate for 24 samples in triplicates, eight standards in duplicates, blank and control in quadrates, excluding samples for the preassessment step (*vide infra*). Some of the wells of the multiplexing plate can be spared for another assay later. However, the controls, blank, and standards will have to be included in each run, which might significantly increase the cost of the experiment. Hence, it is preferable to use the plate all at once. In case some wells were left empty for future use, they must be covered with a sealing tape to avoid cross-contamination during the washing steps.

After preparation and centrifugation, the samples should be kept on ice or stored in the freezer for future use. Spinning down the samples at 13,200 rpm for 10 min at 4°C is usually sufficient to remove cellular debris. Volumes of 12.5 mL of plasma or serum and 50 mL of cell culture supernatant or other biological fluids are required to perform the multiplex assays. The use of magnetic beads and magnetic separation during the various washing steps is usually more convenient and improves reproducibility, as compared to vacuum filtration. This kind of assay can measure up to 500 biomarkers in a single well depending on the available instrument and kits.

The bead component of the kit should be well-suspended, particularly for plexes that contain higher numbers of different conjugated beads (i.e., for capturing different biomarkers). Usually, 30 s are enough time for vortexing, and pipetting should be done from the bottom of the tubes. Furthermore, the beads should be always suspended in the assay buffer and never left dry as they may aggregate. Beads and streptavidin-phycoerythrin (i.e., reporter molecule) are light sensitive and they should be protected from light using aluminum foil.

Although similar principles are usually applied in different laboratory settings, the authors are more familiar with the Bio-Plex 200 System equipped with HTF and a Bio-Plex Pro II Wash Station and the use of magnetic separation rather than using a vacuum manifold.

Procedure:

Eye protection, gloves and universal precautions should be applied, and biosafety level appropriate to the specific samples as recommended by the manufacturer and the institution where the work will be carried out should be considered. Most of these materials should be handled with caution. Materials that can be prepared before starting the assay and some useful hints are provided in Box 4.2 *and* Box 4.3

1. Before starting up the instrument, empty the waste bottle and fill the sheath fluid container.

BOX 4.2 Materials that should be on-site before starting the experiment

Pipettes (well-calibrated, well-trained personnel, careful pipetting, avoid bubbles, and use new pipette tips for every volume transfer).
Multichannel pipettes are important for reducing the duration of the experiment and to improve efficiency.
Aluminum foil, vortex, and centrifuge.
Racks, centrifuge tubes, tips, ice container, calculator.
Kits for calibration, validation, and assays (brought to room temperature).
Media, PBS, or the diluent for standards.

BOX 4.3 General notes

Automatic accessories (e.g., wash station for washing between various steps) save time and improve the accuracy of the measurements.
The diluent of the standard should be similar to the final sample type or matrix. The blank should be the same as the standard diluent.
Do not freeze the kit components.
There should be enough sheath fluid before running the experiment.
Validation should be performed once a month and calibration should be performed before each experiment.
Generally, vortexing, dilutions, and incubation times vary depending on the type of sample and kit in use, and it is important to follow the manufacturer's instructions for maximum accuracy.

2. Start up the instrument and follow the manufacturer's instructions to get it ready for the assay. During the startup procedures, all the assay components and samples should be brought to room temperature.
3. Calibrate and validate the instrument *per* the manufacturer instructions. Ensure that the information in the software protocol matches with the information on the kit components (e.g., lot number, standards concentrations, dilution factors, etc.).
4. Preassessment step (Optional): Assessment of potential adsorption/absorption of biomarkers by the tested materials step is optional and it is described in Section 4.3 (*vide infra*).

5. Vials that contain the lyophilized biomarker standards (i.e., the standard vial) shall be tapped well before opening to avoid materials loss. Reconstitute the standard vial with the recommended buffer (usually the same media used for the samples), vortex and incubate *per* the manufacturer's instructions.
6. Prepare various dilutions from the standards *per* the manufacturer's instructions. Appropriate dilutions are one of the main challenges toward the use of multiplexing techniques, particularly with the higher plexes. It is advisable to prepare the standards, in the same way, every time to minimize variations between the various runs.
7. Prepare the plate layout in the laboratory notebook and in the instrument software protocol (Fig. 4.2). This protocol usually specifies the analytes, assigned wells, instrument settings, and information on the samples, standards, and controls. Adjust all the parameters *per* the manufacturer instructions, which vary depending on several factors (e.g., supplier, type of kit, etc.).
8. The samples are obtained after treatment of cells or animals with the particulate materials (in vitro or in vivo, respectively). They could be tissue culture supernatant, cell or tissue lysates, or serum/plasma that contains the inflammatory mediators or other biomarkers (Fig. 4.3). Centrifugation of samples is important to remove any particulates or debris. Consideration should be taken to avoid potential interference from various ingredients in the samples (e.g., heparin).

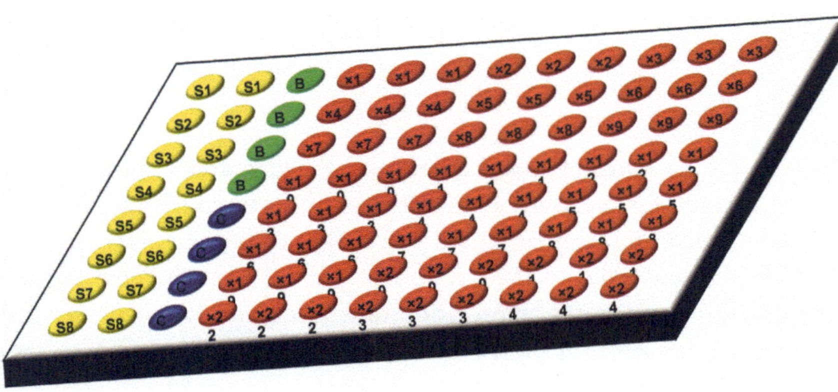

Figure 4.2 Plate layout for the multiplexing experiment. The plate is designed to be carried out in a 96-well plate for 24 samples in triplicates, eight standards in duplicates, blank and control in quadrates, excluding samples for the preassessment step. *Yellow*: standards; *green*: blank, *blue*: controls, and *red*: samples in triplicates from $\times 1$ to $\times 24$.

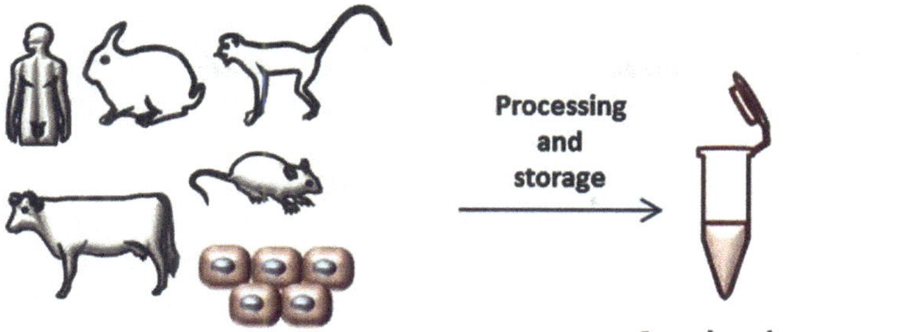

Figure 4.3 Various sources of biological samples. Samples that contain the various biomarkers could be from different biological sources, and usually a small final volume of the processed sample is needed. *Adapted with permission from the Royal Society of Chemistry.*

9. Fill the standards, blank, controls, and samples into a standard 96 well plate (i.e., preplate) as in Fig. 4.2. It is recommended to use slightly higher volumes (e.g., extra 10 μL) than the final volumes (e.g., 50 μL) that will be transferred to the final plate.
10. Samples that contain the inflammatory mediators are then mixed with multiple coded beads for the detection of biomarkers via detection antibodies conjugated onto the surface of the beads (Fig. 4.4). Prepare the conjugated beads in the final plate (i.e., assay plate) and remember that vortexing, spinning down, and wrapping in aluminum foil are critical precautions. Bead preparation is one of the most critical steps throughout the whole experiment, and they must be well suspended as aggregation will compromise the experiment. The color or spectral characteristics of the beads define the type of biomarker.
11. Transfer the content of the preplate into the assay plate after gentle mixing using a multichannel pipette. Remember to change the pipette tips before every new volume transfer.
12. There could be different washing procedures before starting the experiment and between the various steps, depending on the kit and instrument used (follow the manufacturer instructions).
13. Seal the plate with a sealing tape and cover the plate with aluminum foil, shake and incubate. Settings for the shaking and incubation are

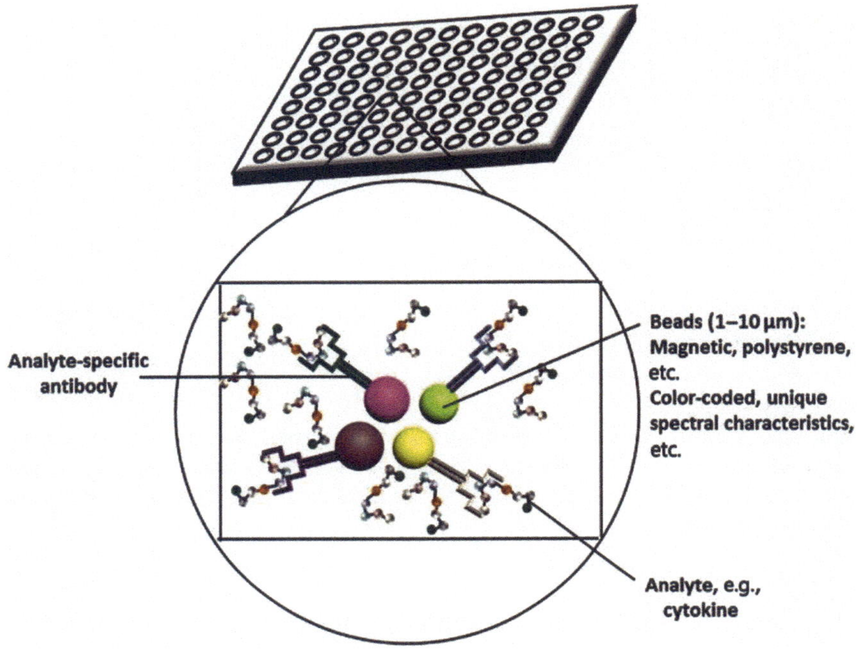

Figure 4.4 Binding of the antibody-conjugated beads to the biomarker. Each bead is conjugated to a specific antibody for binding to a specific analyte. *Adapted with permission from the Royal Society of Chemistry.*

usually provided with the kit. All incubations shall be carried out in the dark (i.e., protected from light by aluminum foil).

14. Slowly remove the sealing tape and remove the buffer from the assay plate and wash *per* the manufacturer's instructions.
15. After a series of washes, biotinylated-antibody is added to bind to the biomarker-detection antibody complex on a secondary site of the biomarker to form sandwich-like complexes. Quick spin the antibody before pipetting and start this step during the incubation of samples with the conjugated beads. Sometimes, detection antibodies need to be prepared 10 min before use. Repeat steps 13 and 14.
16. Warm up the instrument.
17. Streptavidin-phycoerythrin conjugate is then added to form the final detection complexes in quantities that are correlated with the biomarker concentrations (Fig. 4.5). Quick spin the streptavidin-phycoerythrin conjugate before pipetting, protect from light and start this step during the incubation with the biotinylated antibody

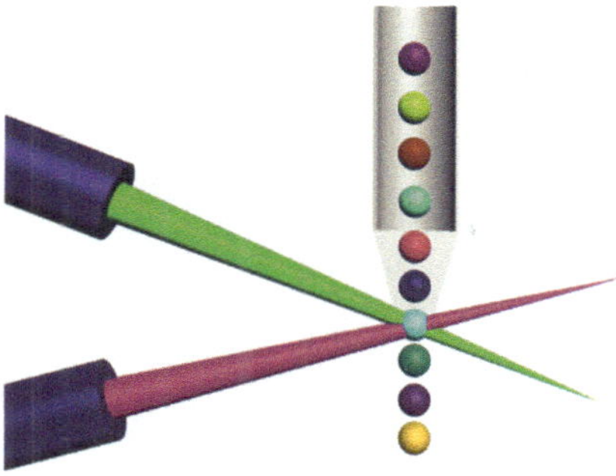

Figure 4.5 The color or spectral characteristics of the beads define the type of biomarker. The final detection complexes are formed in quantities that are correlated with the biomarker concentration. *Adapted with permission from the Royal Society of Chemistry.*

(step 15). Streptavidin-phycoerythrin might (Elsabahy & Wooley, 2013) need to be prepared 10 min before use. Repeat steps 13 and 14.

18. Resuspend in the assay buffer, seal the plate, cover the plate with aluminum foil, and shake *per* the manufacturer's instructions. Remove sealing tape and any bubbles from the samples before loading them into the instrument.

19. Sometimes, it is possible to rerun the plate in case any problem was encountered during the first run. However, this should be done carefully *per* the manufacturer's instructions as the original data may be rewritten.

20. Instrument shut down and maintenance should be performed *per* the manufacturer's instructions.

4.3 Preassessment step: optional

Biomarkers may be adsorbed on the surfaces and/or absorbed within internal regions of micro or nanoparticles (Elsabahy & Wooley, 2013; Hussain et al., 2009; Kocbach et al., 2008; Val et al., 2009; Veranth et al., 2007). This interference reduces the available concentrations of the biomarkers, thereby leading to potential artifacts and data misinterpretation (Fig. 4.6). The extent of interference depends on the nature of the

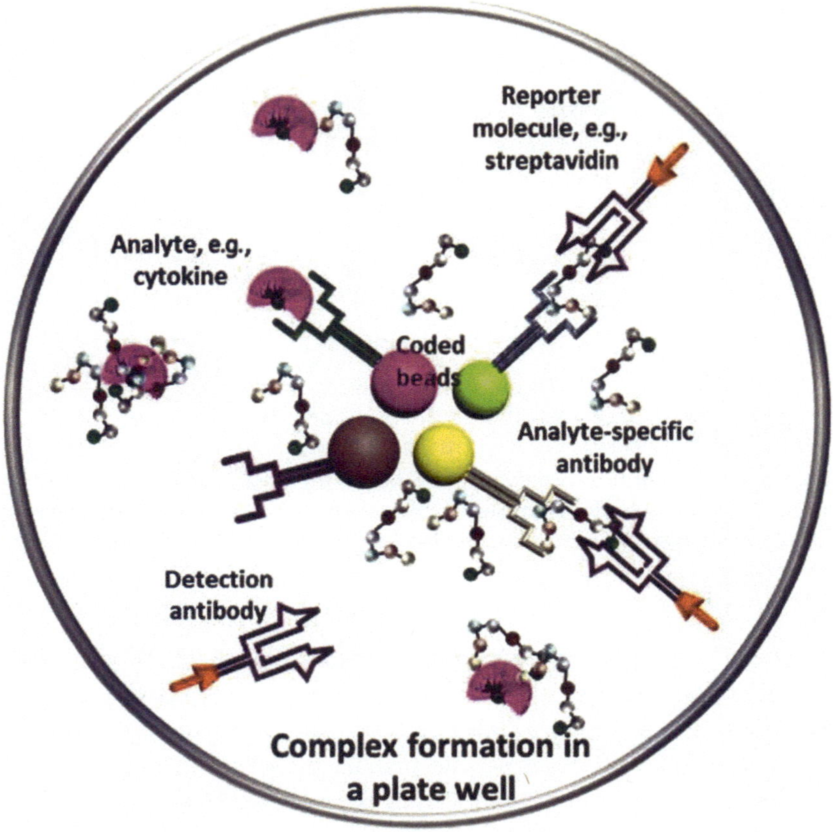

Figure 4.6 Possible interference of nanomaterials with the kit components during the multiplexing assay. Analytes may be adsorbed on the surface of the particulate materials or absorbed within their internal regions. *Adapted with permission from Elsevier.*

biomarker and the physicochemical characteristics of the tested materials. Recently, we have reported on the necessity for a reassessment of nanomaterials immunotoxicity due to the potential interactions between nanoparticles and biomarkers during the multiplexing assay (Elsabahy & Wooley, 2018), which has not been carefully assessed in previous studies. The assessment of interference can be carried out independently or using multiplexing assays. Away from the multiplexing experiments, the intracellular and released proteins and mRNA expression levels may be measured, although potential interference from the tested materials might also exist. Alternatively, biomarker standards can be premixed with various concentrations of the tested materials. Then, the measured concentrations are compared with the same biomarker concentrations in the absence of the tested materials.

Procedure:

1. Mix 200 μL of the stock standard solution (standard lyophilized powder reconstituted in 500 μL of diluent) and 3800 μL of the media. Dilute the formed solution twice with the media (i.e., 40 × dilution of the stock standard solution).
2. Prepare 250 μL-fractions of the finally prepared solution.
3. Add 50 μL of media (i.e., control biomarkers with no interference) to one of the 250 μL fraction and 50 μL of the tested materials or various concentrations of the tested materials to the other 250 μL fractions.
4. Run the assay as previously described and compare the concentrations of the biomarkers in the standard solutions mixed with the tested materials relative to the concentrations of the biomarkers in absence of the tested materials (i.e., fractions mixed with the media).
5. Concentrations of the tested materials that interfere with the assay (i.e., reduce the available biomarker measured concentrations) should be excluded from the assay or accounted for during the analysis. It is expected that for materials that interfere with the assay, this interference will increase upon increasing the concentration of the tested materials.

4.4 Data mining and analysis

Data output is usually presented as median fluorescence intensity and concentration (pg/mL). The outliers should be removed before data analysis. This can be done manually or automatically depending on the software. Negative values might be due to a lower amount (or absence) of analyte or due to an effect of the sample matrix. Remember that the blank values are usually subtracted automatically from the resultant values of all other assay wells.

References

Elsabahy, M., & Wooley, K. L. (2013). Cytokines as biomarkers of nanoparticle immunotoxicity. *Chemical Society Reviews, 42*(12), 5552–5576. Available from https://doi.org/10.1039/c3cs60064e.

Elsabahy, M., & Wooley, K. L. (2015). Data mining as a guide for the construction of cross-linked nanoparticles with low immunotoxicity via control of polymer chemistry and supramolecular assembly. *Accounts of Chemical Research*, *48*(6), 1620–1630. Available from https://doi.org/10.1021/acs.accounts.5b00066.

Elsabahy, M., & Wooley, K. L. (2018). Reassessment of nanomaterials immunotoxicity. *Nano Today*, *20*, 10–12. Available from https://doi.org/10.1016/j.nantod.2018.01.002.

Elsabahy, M., Heo, G. S., Lim, S. M., Sun, G., & Wooley, K. L. (2015). Polymeric nanostructures for imaging and therapy. *Chemical Reviews*, *115*(19), 10967–11011. Available from https://doi.org/10.1021/acs.chemrev.5b00135.

Elsabahy, M., Li, A., Zhang, F., Sultan, D., Liu, Y., & Wooley, K. L. (2013). Differential immunotoxicities of poly(ethylene glycol)- vs. poly(carboxybetaine)-coated nanoparticles. *Journal of Controlled Release*, *172*(3), 641–652. Available from https://doi.org/10.1016/j.jconrel.2013.09.010.

Hussain, S., Boland, S., Baeza-Squiban, A., Hamel, R., Thomassen, L. C. J., Martens, J. A., Billon-Galland, M. A., Fleury-Feith, J., Moisan, F., Pairon, J. C., & Marano, F. (2009). Oxidative stress and proinflammatory effects of carbon black and titanium dioxide nanoparticles: Role of particle surface area and internalized amount. *Toxicology*, *260*(1–3), 142–149. Available from https://doi.org/10.1016/j.tox.2009.04.001.

Jani, D., Allinson, J., Berisha, F., Cowan, K. J., Devanarayan, V., Gleason, C., Jeromin, A., Keller, S., Khan, M. U., Nowatzke, B., Rhyne, P., & Stephen, L. (2016). Recommendations for use and fit-for-purpose validation of biomarker multiplex ligand binding assays in drug development. *AAPS Journal*, *18*(1), 1–14. Available from https://doi.org/10.1208/s12248-015-9820-y.

Kocbach, A., Totlandsdal, A. I., Låg, M., Refsnes, M., & Schwarze, P. E. (2008). Differential binding of cytokines to environmentally relevant particles: A possible source for misinterpretation of in vitro results? *Toxicology Letters*, *176*(2), 131–137. Available from https://doi.org/10.1016/j.toxlet.2007.10.014.

Mao, L., Liu, Y., Yang, S., Li, Y., Zhang, X., & Wei, Y. (2019). Recent advances and progress of fluorescent bio-/chemosensors based on aggregation-induced emission molecules. *Dyes and Pigments*, *162*, 611–623. Available from https://doi.org/10.1016/j.dyepig.2018.10.045.

Mitragotri, S., Lammers, T., Bae, Y. H., Schwendeman, S., De Smedt, S., Leroux, J. C., Peer, D., Kwon, I. C., Harashima, H., Kikuchi, A., Oh, Y. K., Torchilin, V., Hennink, W., Hanes, J., & Park, K. (2017). Drug delivery research for the future: Expanding the nano horizons and beyond. *Journal of Controlled Release*, *246*, 183–184. Available from https://doi.org/10.1016/j.jconrel.2017.01.011.

Mohamed, N. K., Hamad, M. A., Hafez, M. Z. E., Wooley, K. L., & Elsabahy, M. (2017). Nanomedicine in management of hepatocellular carcinoma: Challenges and opportunities. *International Journal of Cancer*, *140*(7), 1475–1484. Available from https://doi.org/10.1002/ijc.30517.

Shi, J., Deng, Q., Wan, C., Zheng, M., Huang, F., & Tang, B. (2017). Fluorometric probing of the lipase level as acute pancreatitis biomarkers based on interfacially controlled aggregation-induced emission (AIE). *Chemical Science*, *8*(9), 6188–6195. Available from https://doi.org/10.1039/c7sc02189e.

Val, S., Hussain, S., Boland, S., Hamel, R., Baeza-Squiban, A., & Marano, F. (2009). Carbon black and titanium dioxide nanoparticles induce pro-inflammatory responses in bronchial epithelial cells: Need for multiparametric evaluation due to adsorption artifacts. *Inhalation Toxicology*, *21*(1), 115–122. Available from https://doi.org/10.1080/08958370902942533.

Veranth, J. M., Kaser, E. G., Veranth, M. M., Koch, M., & Yost, G. S. (2007). Cytokine responses of human lung cells (BEAS-2B) treated with micron-sized and nanoparticles

of metal oxides compared to soil dusts. *Particle and Fibre Toxicology*, *4*. Available from https://doi.org/10.1186/1743-8977-4-2.
Zhang, X., Zhang, X., Yang, B., Liu, M., Liu, W., Chen, Y., & Wei, Y. (2014). Polymerizable aggregation-induced emission dye-based fluorescent nanoparticles for cell imaging applications. *Polymer Chemistry*, *5*(2), 356–360. Available from https://doi.org/10.1039/c3py01226c.

CHAPTER 5

Recommendations and use of multiplex biomarker assays

Paul W. Rhyne
Bill & Melinda Gates Medical Research Institute, Cambridge, MA, United States

5.1 Introduction

Immunoassays are commonly used tools to measure many different types of analytes, including biomarkers and biologic-based drugs. Most immunoassays rely on antibodies as critical reagents to capture and detect the analyte of interest in a biological matrix. However, ligand binding molecules that bind to one another can be used in lieu of antibodies. Thus the industry has applied the term ligand binding assays (LBAs) to encompass a broader range of assay formats. Traditionally, assays are designed to detect the presence of a single analyte as a "singleplex" assay. There are a wide variety of detection technologies used to build ligand binding assays that include enzyme-driven detection, chemiluminescence, radioactive isotopes, fluorescence, and electrochemiluminescence. There are now many technologies that allow singleplex LBAs to be combined and used to measure their respective analyte in a simultaneous manner in a single reaction vessel. Performing multiple assays together in a single reaction vessel in this context is referred to as multiplexing. In contrast, technologies that take a sample and portion it into multiple single reaction vessels each containing a singleplex assay would not be categorized as multiplexing in this chapter as the assays are performed separately from one another.

The biggest advantage of multiplexed assays is the efficiency of sample analysis. This efficiency includes a reduction in labor and time versus conducting each of the assays separately. In situations where sample availability is limited, multiplexed assays would make the most use of the sample in comparison to a series of singleplex assays. Manufacturers of commercial singleplex assays have recognized the utility of multiplex assays by combining their singleplex assays into a multiplexed assay.

Multiplexing technologies typically rely on either microbead or solid-phase planar array-based platforms that require specialized instruments.

Immunomodulatory Effects of Nanomaterials
DOI: https://doi.org/10.1016/B978-0-323-90604-3.00006-1

Bead-based technologies typically distinguish LBAs from one another by assigning a uniquely identified bead set to each assay in contrast to solid-phase planar arrays that distinguish each LBA by a unique location on the solid phase surface. Detection of captured analytes from each assay varies between technology platforms but often uses fluorescence, chemiluminescence, or electrochemiluminescence. Several recent publications comprehensively review the latest multiplexing technologies (Hsu et al., 2009; Ling et al., 2007; Marquette et al., 2012; Tighe et al., 2013).

There are some considerations in evaluating multiplexed assays to ensure that they will meet the needs of the study. These include the range of detection, reference standards, selectivity, specificity, and sensitivity. Although there are many advantages offered by multiplexing, there are unique issues and challenges singleplex assays do not encounter. It is important to understand that multiplexed assays are optimized to ensure all the assays work well together. This may be different than the optimal assay conditions for each assay run independently. Thus the performance of each assay may be different in a multiplexed assay than in a singleplex format.

5.1.1 Evaluation of multiplex assays

5.1.1.1 Selecting the right size of multiplex assay

Multiplexing is designed to make sample analysis more efficient by generating data on many analytes without increasing labor and conserving samples. Ultimately, the number of analytes in each multiplex assay is determined by the intended use of the data. There are situations where scientists are using multiplexed assays for discovery such as looking for biological patterns or relative differences between the analytes. In this case, a large plex with lower performance characteristics may be acceptable. However, if the multiplex assay is to be used to quantitate each analyte and the resulting data are used to support more critical decisions, a smaller more defined multiplex assay with better performance would be the better choice. Consider a situation when one of the multiplexed assays fails to perform. Repeating the analysis for that one analyte is more costly with a large plex assay versus a smaller plex assay. With regards to validation, a multiplex assay with a smaller number of analytes is easier to do than a multiplex assay with a larger number of analytes. Ultimately, the decision on the number of analytes in an assay is a balance between the quality of the data and the other benefits of multiplexing, such as savings on matrix volume, time, and cost.

5.1.1.2 Effects of sample matrix

Ligand binding assays are usually developed in buffer environments, which is different from measuring the analyte in clinical samples that often contain analytes with similar or shared epitopes, soluble receptors, rheumatoid factor, heterophilic antibodies, or other molecules that can interfere with the assay (Todd et al., 2011). These factors are often referred to as "matrix" effects. The reported performance characteristics of a multiplex assay may be based on experiments done in assay buffer as opposed to sample matrix such as serum or plasma. Thus the reported assay performance may be different when the assay is applied to samples. A common method to assess matrix effects is to measure purified versions of the analyte spiked into a biological or clinical sample. Purified proteins are often different than the native forms in many ways including glycosylation, phosphorylation, sequence differences, and tertiary structures. Thus these experiments may not reflect the measurement of endogenous forms found in the samples. With these considerations, it is important to evaluate multiplex assays using a sample of the same matrix as the intended samples to ensure the assay will deliver results.

Parallelism may be an option to assess the influence of matrix on the assay if existing samples containing high enough levels of the analyte are available. Parallelism using incurred individual subject samples that have high levels of the analytes is ideal. However, if these samples are not available, commercially purchased individual samples can also be used. Establishing parallelism for a multiplex assay follows the same guidelines as a single analyte assay. Parallelism also assists in determining the minimum, and possibly maximum, sample dilution factor that can be used in the assay.

5.1.1.3 Reproducibility

In a multiplexing environment, the precision of each assay will likely vary from the same assay run in a singleplex format. The best way to assess precision is to use a quality control (QC) panel made from a set of samples that contain the analytes of interest covering the target range of study samples. It is unlikely that any one sample will contain all the analytes in the multiplex panel. Thus some QC samples would be used for some analytes and not others. The QC panel would also be used to monitor assay performance during sample analysis after validation is successfully completed. Precision of the multiplex assay should be determined using this set of QC samples, and the acceptance criteria should be based on the intended use and biological variability of the population with the expected physiological changes taken into account.

5.1.1.4 Lot-to-lot variability

One of the most critical aspects of multiplex assays is making them reproducible across multiple lots. Lot-to-lot variability is often related to critical reagents for one or more analytes, for example, the quality of recombinant proteins, the capture or detection reagents, and a general lack of critical reagent characterization. Commercially purchased multiplexed assays are subject to unannounced changes in critical kit components, overall poor kit quality, and expiration dates on kits or individual components associated with the kit lot during the study. Some manufacturers will create new lots of a multiplex assay by mixing preexisting and new singleplex assays together, making lot-to-lot consistency more difficult to control. Control strategies for subsequent lots and changes to critical reagents should be put into place to improve consistency as much as possible. A large QC panel consisting of a set of individual samples (>20) is a good way to evaluate lot-to-lot variability. Prequalification of each new lot is done using the QC panel where the new lot is compared to the existing lot to assess lot differences. Changes in critical reagents should also be prequalified using a similar strategy. If there is significant variability between lots (as defined by the lab), the user can either look for alternate lots or devise a statistical strategy to bridge the data between two lots. Laboratories that expect to use the assay over a long period of time should try to secure assays from a single lot and pre-qualify new lots as much as possible. Thus for multiplex assays, an early assessment of the number of kits required to cover validation and sample analysis is highly recommended.

5.1.2 Unique challenges with multiplexed assays

5.1.2.1 Finding the best sample dilution scheme

Samples will likely require some level of dilution to ensure high levels of analytes fall within the range of detection or to mitigate the effects of the sample matrix on the assay. Determining the best sample dilution to use should consider the concentrations of all analytes present in the sample. It is not uncommon for a given sample to have low concentrations of some of the analytes and high concentrations of others, which limits the amount of dilution to ensure all the analytes fall into the detection range. Alternatively, each sample can be run at multiple dilutions to ensure all the analytes fall into their quantitative range. Thus multiplexing often requires a compromise in sample dilution that may not be optimal for every analyte being measured. This is further compounded by changes in the analyte concentration that may occur with treatment or disease. If an acceptable sample dilution cannot be achieved for all the analytes, the samples will need to run at different dilutions. The last option is to remove the problematic analytes from the multiplex panel and run them separately.

A common technique to determine the best sample dilution scheme is to run a set of individual samples, preferably target or disease-state samples, over a range of dilutions. The variability of the sample replicates should be analyzed to ensure that they are within the desired acceptable variability for the assay. The sample dilution scheme that yields acceptable reproducibility is selected for the assay. The addition of blocking reagents, detergents, heterophilic antibody blockers, etc. may also be tested as they often help mitigate matrix effects.

5.1.2.2 Cross-reactivity in multiplexed assays

Ligand binding assays often have capture or detection reagents that bind to similar epitopes on other analytes present in the sample. This will lead to cross-reactive binding to these analytes and either interfere with the detection of the intended analyte or give a false positive signal if both capture and reporter binding ligands cross-react. Unfortunately, multiplexed assays amplify this situation by increasing the number of critical capture and detection reagents in the assay. This creates an environment that is more susceptible to cross-reactivity issues than singleplex assays. One method to assess cross-reactivity is to analyze one analyte at a time in the multiplexed assay so that the only signal generated is in the appropriate assay. Alternatively, a mixture of the analytes minus one can be tested so that all the assays generate a signal except the one missing the analyte. Another option is to compare the multiplex assay results to a well-characterized singleplex assay (Backen et al., 2014; Bastarache et al., 2014; Salvante et al., 2012) and demonstrate comparable results. Cross-reactivity in multiplexed assays should be assessed to ensure that the interpretation of results is accurate. The higher the plex, the more likely cross-reactivity will become an issue.

5.1.2.3 Challenges of crosstalk

Multiplexing technologies rely on signals from all the assays being generated at the same time. Sometimes these signals can spread into the adjacent well, spot, or bead leading to "carryover," "bleed-over," "blooming," or "leaching" events where the measured analytes in adjacent wells or beads yield inflated measurements. Multiplex technologies should have a mechanism to identify crosstalk and provide a solution to mitigate these effects. Experiments can be set up to test for crosstalk by varying the concentration of one analyte over the full dynamic range of the assay while keeping the other analytes at very low concentrations. Blank samples or samples missing one or more analytes can also be used to reveal increased background signals caused by crosstalk. If crosstalk becomes problematic, the scientist will need to decide if the multiplex assay can be used or not. One solution is to characterize or define conditions where crosstalk interferes with the assay and review the results accordingly to identify problematic data.

5.1.2.4 Fit for purpose validation of multiplex assays

Data generated by multiplexed assays will be used in many ways including basic research, drug development, clinical biomarker measurement, and diagnostics. This in turn leads to a wide range of how the data will be used and analyzed between the different laboratories. In some cases, the data will be used to support clinical studies while in others the data may be used for hypothesis generation in academic research. Depending on how the data are used, the assays should undergo some level of assay validation before the data are generated. In some circumstances, the assays should be characterized by a rigorous amount of analytical performance to ensure the reliability of the data for its intended use. While in other circumstances such as hypothesis generation, the analytical performance of the assay is less important. There are many excellent publications that provide guidance on how to validate assays and how to ensure that the analytical performance is fit for its intended purpose (Chau et al., 2008; Lee et al., 2005, 2006), as well as the recent draft guidance for industry on bioanalytical method validation (Guidance for Industry: Bioanalytical Method Validation, 2018). There are also publications that describe how to perform a fit-for-purpose validation of commercial kits (Bowsher & Sailstad, 2008; Fraser & Soderstrom, 2014) and commercial multiplex kits (Backen et al., 2009; Belabani et al., 2013; Chowdhury et al., 2009; Jani et al., 2016; Li et al., 2012). Most of these recommendations apply equally to singleplex and multiplex assays. Validation of multiplexed assays should include an assessment of cross-reactivity and crosstalk as described earlier. In essence, the assays should be validated to a level to ensure the performance and data integrity are suitable for the intended use.

5.1.2.5 Assay sensitivity

Assays regardless of single- or multiplexed will have a limit on the amount of analyte they can reliably detect in a sample. This applies to both the low concentrations and high concentrations in a sample. These limits are defined as the upper and lower limit of quantitation (ULOQ and LLOQ, respectively). Determining the limits of quantitation for multiplex assays is essentially the same process as used in singleplex assays. Basically, the analyte is to be tested at a range of concentrations in the target matrix. The upper and lower limits of quantitation are the concentrations that generate measurable results within acceptable assay precision limits. In the multiplexed assay, the LLOQ and ULOQ should be tested separately and in the presence of all the analytes to ensure that these limits are not influenced by the other analytes. The estimated LLOQ and ULOQ are then used to define the range of quantitation for the assay.

5.2 Conclusions

Multiplex assays are very powerful analytical tools that are widely used across the scientific community. Multiplex assays have the same challenges and issues that singleplex assays have, but also have unique challenges due to the more complex environment. These unique challenges include altered detection ranges, diminished sensitivity, crosstalk, and increased opportunity for cross-reactivity. However, these unique challenges can be characterized and overcome with the right strategy. Multiplexing assays can be quite effective at increasing the speed of analysis and providing large data sets while minimizing sample size. Many multiplexed assays have been designed and built to meet the stringent requirements of diagnostic assay approval including the technology and software to support the assay.

The application of multiplexed assays to complex biological problems has improved the ability to diagnose and understand diseases to enable better treatment and human health. For example, a panel of biomarkers was designed to generate a disease score for rheumatoid arthritis patients, which is predictive of radiographic damage (Curtis et al., 2019). Diagnostic multiplexed assays to help physicians identify underlying viral pathogens in respiratory infections (Diaz-Decaro et al., 2018; Leber et al., 2020; Pabbaraju et al., 2011), which in turn helps patient treatment. Progressive neurological diseases such as Alzheimer's disease are being investigated with panels of multiplexed biomarkers to predict the progression of Alzheimer's disease and identify potential new biomarkers (Kang et al., 2012; Moon et al., 2021;

Slaets et al., 2014). Immunogenicity assays have been multiplexed together to not only detect the presence of antibodies directed against the therapeutic but also isotype reactive antibodies all in the same assay (Alleyn et al., 2020). Complex human diseases will likely require more in-depth biomarker analysis to better understand the biology of these diseases and develop treatments that improve outcomes.

The additional challenges that multiplexed assays described in this chapter can be dealt with in an effective manner. The continued improvement of technologies and better characterization of critical reagents will improve the performance of multiplexed assays. Multiplexing is a powerful scientific tool that provides faster more efficient analysis and will continue to be a significant factor in improving human health.

References

Alleyn, M., Closson, K., Gentile, A., Gulbis, N., Taylor, C., & Rhyne, P. (2020). Design and evaluation of a multiplexed assay to assess human immunogenicity against Humira®. *The AAPS Journal, 22*(5), 104–116.

Backen, A., Renehan, A., Clamp, A., Berzuini, C., Zhou, C., Oza, A., Bannoo, S., Scherer, S., Banks, R., Dive, C., & Jayson, G. (2014). The combination of circulating Ang1 and Tie2 levels predicts progression-free survival advantage in bevacizumab-treated patients with ovarian cancer. *Clinical Cancer Research: An Official Journal of the American Association for Cancer Research, 20*(17), 4549–4558.

Backen, A. C., Cummings, J., Mitchell, C., Jayson, G., Ward, T., & Dive, C. (2009). 'Fit-for-purpose' validation of searchlight multiplex ELISAs of angiogenesis for clinical trial use. *Journal of Immunological Methods, 342*(1–2), 106–114.

Bastarache, J. A., Koyama, T., Wickersham, N., & Ware, L. (2014). Validation of a multiplex electrochemiluminescent immunoassay platform in human and mouse samples. *Journal of Immunological Methods, 408*, 13–23.

Belabani, C., Rajasekharan, S., Poupon, V., Johnson, T., & Bar-Or, A. (2013). A condensed performance-validation strategy for multiplex detection kits used in studies of human clinical samples. *Journal of Immunological Methods, 387*(1–2), 1–10.

Bowsher, R. R., & Sailstad, J. M. (2008). Insights in the application of research-grade diagnostic kits for biomarker assessments in support of clinical drug development: bioanalysis of circulating concentrations of soluble receptor activator of nuclear factor ligand. *Journal of Pharmaceutical and Biomedical Analysis, 48*(5), 1282–1289.

Chau, C., Rixie, O., McLeod, H., & Figg, W. (2008). Validation of analytic method for biomarkers used in drug development. *Clinical Cancer Research, 14*(19), 5967–5976.

Chowdhury, F., Williams, A., & Johnson, P. (2009). Validation and comparison of two multiplex technologies, Luminex® and Mesoscale Discovery, for human cytokine profiling. *Journal of Immunological Methods, 340*(1), 55–64.

Curtis, J. R., Brahe, C. H., Østergaard, M., Lund Hetland, M., Hambardzumyan, K., Saevarsdottir, S., Wang, X., Flake, D. D., II, Sasso, E. H., & Huizinga, T. W. (2019). Predicting risk for radiographic damage in rheumatoid arthritis: Comparative analysis of the multi-biomarker disease activity score and conventional measures of disease activity in multiple studies. *Current Medical Research and Opinion, 35*(9), 1483–1493.

Diaz-Decaro, J., Green, N., & Godwin, H. (2018). Critical evaluation of FDA-approved respiratory multiplex assays for public health surveillance. *Expert Review of Molecular Diagnostics*, *18*(7), 631–643.

Fraser, S., & Soderstrom, C. (2014). Due diligence in the characterization of matrix effects in a total IL-13 Singulex™ method. *Bioanalysis*, *6*(8), 1123–1129.

Guidance for Industry: Bioanalytical Method Validation. (2018). U.S. Department of Health and Human Services Food and Drug Administration Center for Drug Evaluation and Research (CDER), Center for Veterinary Medicine (CVM).

Hsu, H. Y., Joos, T. O., & Koga, H. (2009). Multiplex microsphere-based flow cytometric platforms for protein analysis and their application in clinical proteomics – from assays to results. *Electrophoresis*, *30*(23), 4008–4019.

Jani, D., Allinson, J., Berisha, F., Cowan, K., Devanarayan, V., Gleason, C., Jeromin, A., Keller, S., Khan, M., Nowatzke, B., Rhyne, P., & Stephen, L. (2016). Recommendations for use and fit-for-purpose validation of biomarker multiplex ligand binding assays in drug development. *The AAPS Journal*, *18*(1), 1–14.

Kang, J. H., Vanderstichele, H., Trojanowski, J. Q., & Shaw, L. M. (2012). Simultaneous analysis of cerebrospinal fluid biomarkers using microsphere-based xMAP multiplex technology for early detection of Alzheimer's disease. *Methods (San Diego, Calif.)*, *56*(4), 484–493.

Leber, A. L., Lisby, J. G., Hansen, G., Relich, R. F., Schneider, U. V., Granato, P., Young, S., Pareja, J., & Hannet, I. (2020). Multicenter evaluation of the QIAstat-Dx respiratory panel for detection of viruses and bacteria in nasopharyngeal swab specimens. *Journal of Clinical Microbiology*, *58*(5), e00155-20.

Lee, J. W., Devanarayan, V., Barrett, Y. C., Weiner, R., Allinson, J., Fountain, S., Keller, S., Weinryb, I., Green, M., Duan, L., Rogers, J. A., Millham, R., O'Brien, P. J., Sailstad, J., Khan, M., Ray, C., & Wagner, J. A. (2006). Fit-for-purpose method development and validation for successful biomarker measurement. *Pharmaceutical Research*, *23*(2), 312–328.

Lee, J. W., Weiner, R. S., Sailstad, J. M., Bowsher, R. R., Knuth, D. W., O'Brien, P. J., Fourcroy, J. L., Dixit, R., Pandite, L., Pietrusko, R. G., Soares, H. D., Quarmby, V., Vesterqvist, O. L., Potter, D. M., Witliff, J. L., Fritche, H. A., O'Leary, T., Perlee, L., Kadam, S., & Wagner, J. A. (2005). Method validation and measurement of biomarkers in nonclinical and clinical samples in drug development: a conference report. *Pharmaceutical Research*, *22*(4), 499–511.

Li, D., Chiu, H., Gupta, V., & Chan, D. (2012). Validation of a multiplex immunoassay for serum angiogenic factors as biomarkers for aggressive prostate cancer. *Clinica Chimica Acta*, *413*(0), 1506–1511.

Ling, M. M., Ricks, C., & Lea, P. (2007). Multiplexing molecular diagnostics and immunoassays using emerging microarray technologies. *Expert Review of Molecular Diagnostics*, 7(1), 87–98.

Marquette, C. A., Corgier, B. P., & Blum, L. J. (2012). Recent advances in multiplex immunoassays. *Bioanalysis*, *4*(8), 927–936.

Moon, S., Kim, S., Mankhong, S., Choi, S. H., Vandijck, M., Kostanjevecki, V., Jeong, J. H., Yoon, S. J., Park, K. W., Kim, E. J., Yoon, B., Kim, H. J., Jang, J. W., Hong, J. Y., Park, D. H., Shaw, L. M., & Kang, J. H. (2021). Alzheimer's cerebrospinal biomarkers from Lumipulse fully automated immunoassay: concordance with amyloid-beta PET and manual immunoassay in Koreans: CSF AD biomarkers measured by Lumipulse in Koreans. *Alzheimer's Research & Therapy*, *13*(1), 22–34.

Pabbaraju, K., Wong, S., Lee, B., Tellier, R., Fonseca, K., Louie, M., & Drews, S. J. (2011). Comparison of a singleplex real-time RT-PCR assay and multiplex respiratory viral panel assay for detection of influenza "A" in respiratory specimens. *Influenza and Other Respiratory Viruses*, *5*(2), 99–103.

Salvante, K. G., Brindle, E., McConnell, D., & O'Connor, P.A., K. (2012). Nepomnaschy Validation of a new multiplex assay against individual immunoassays for the quantification of reproductive, stress, and energetic metabolism biomarkers in urine specimens. *American Journal of Human Biology: The Official Journal of the Human Biology Council*, *24*(1), 81–86.

Slaets, S., Vanmechelen, E., Le Bastard, N., Decraemer, H., Vandijck, M., Martin, J., De Deyn, P., & Engelborghs, S. (2014). Increased CSF α-synuclein levels in Alzheimer's disease: correlation with tau levels. *Alzheimer's & Dementia: the Journal of the Alzheimer's Association*, *10*(5 Suppl.), S290–S298.

Tighe, P., Negm, O., Todd, I., & Fairclough, L. (2013). Utility, reliability, and reproducibility of immunoassay multiplex kits. *Methods (San Diego, Calif.)*, *61*(1), 23–29.

Todd, D. J., Knowlton, N., Amato, M., Frank, M. B., Schur, P. H., Izmailova, E. S., Roubenoff, R., Shadick, N. A., Weinblatt, M. E., Centola, M., & Lee, D. M. (2011). Erroneous augmentation of multiplex assay measurements in patients with rheumatoid arthritis due to heterophilic binding by serum rheumatoid factor. *Arthritis and Rheumatism*, *63*(4), 894–903.

CHAPTER 6

Precautions during evaluation of immunotoxicity of particulate materials*

Mahmoud Elsabahy[1,2,3] **and Karen L. Wooley**[2]
[1]School of Biotechnology and Science Academy, Badr University in Cairo, Badr City, Cairo, Egypt
[2]Department of Chemistry, Laboratory for Synthetic-Biologic Interactions, Texas A&M University, College Station, TX, United States
[3]Department of Pharmaceutics, Faculty of Pharmacy, Assiut University, Assiut, Egypt

There is an increasing interest in the use of nanosized materials for a diversity of biomedical applications. There are several nanosized therapeutics and diagnostics on the market, in different phases of clinical trials, or undergoing rigorous investigation in several laboratories for potential treatment and diagnosis of numerous diseases (Elsabahy et al., 2015). Safety remains a critical issue in the clinical use of nano- and biotechnology-based products. Evaluating overexpression of proinflammatory cytokines in response to treatment with newly developed materials is among the various tools for in vitro and in vivo preclinical and clinical screening of biomaterials (Dobrovolskaia & McNeil, 2007; Elsabahy & Wooley, 2013, 2015). This chapter describes technical procedures to allow for the generation of accurate data, free from artifacts, for the precise and accurate evaluation of immunotoxicity of nanomaterials during multiplexing assays.

Cytokines have a major role in regulating the immune system, and they are commonly measured to explore the effects of biomaterials on the immune system and may also provide partial prediction on the in vivo pharmacokinetics and biodistribution of nanomaterials (Elsabahy et al., 2013; Hunter & Jones, 2015; O'Shea et al., 2002). Enzyme-linked immunosorbent assay and, more recently, multiplex arrays are among the most commonly utilized techniques for measurements of cytokines and

* Adapted with permission from Elsabahy, M., & Wooley, K. L. (2018). Reassessment of nanomaterials immunotoxicity. *Nano Today, 20*, 10–12. https://doi.org/10.1016/j.nantod.2018.01.002.

Immunomodulatory Effects of Nanomaterials
DOI: https://doi.org/10.1016/B978-0-323-90604-3.00001-2

inflammatory mediators, both in vitro and in vivo. Multiplexing technologies have reduced the required analysis times and sample sizes and have allowed simultaneous analyses of up to hundreds of biomarkers in a few microliter sample volumes, with high sensitivity and accuracy. Although the selection of the technique for quantifying cytokine levels, sometimes, depends on the available instrumentation on site, a focus is being given here on the technologies that utilize capture antibodies immobilized on microspheres for multianalyte profiling.

There are several procedures involved in the in vitro multiplexing analysis. Firstly, nanomaterials are incubated with cells for predetermined time intervals. After incubation, tissue culture supernatant, cell or tissue lysates are mixed with multiple coded beads for detection of biomarkers via detection antibodies conjugated onto the surface of the beads. Then, after a series of washes to remove the unbound cytokines, biotinylated-antibody is added to bind to the cytokine-detection antibody complex on a secondary site of the cytokine, to form a sandwich-like complex. A reporter molecule (e.g., streptavidin-phycoerythrin conjugate) is then added to generate the final detection complexes in quantities that are correlated with the cytokine concentration; whereas, the color or spectral characteristics of the beads themselves define the type of cytokine.

There are several limitations associated with the multiplexing techniques, and important factors to be considered, such as variations in the detection limit and half-lives of cytokines, cross-reactivity, lot-to-lot variability, validation, calibration, handling, presence of endogenous or exogenous materials that may interfere with the analysis and complex formation, etc. An excellent review has been published recently by the AAPS Biomarker Discussion group on solutions for some of the challenges toward the appropriate use of multiplexing techniques for drug development and fit-for-purpose-based validation (Jani et al., 2016). However, potential interactions between cytokines and nanomaterials have been overlooked, and there are no reports available on preassessment of these potential interactions during the multiplex assays. These interactions may result in artifacts and data misinterpretation, due to reductions in the available concentrations of cytokines for analysis or interfering with the formation of cytokine–antibody complexes (Fig. 6.1). Adsorption of cytokines on different types of nanoparticles (e.g., carbon and titanium dioxide, and polymeric nanoparticles) has been observed previously, and adsorption extent depended on the nature of the cytokines and nanoparticles (Elsabahy et al., 2013; Hussain et al., 2009; Kocbach et al., 2008; Val

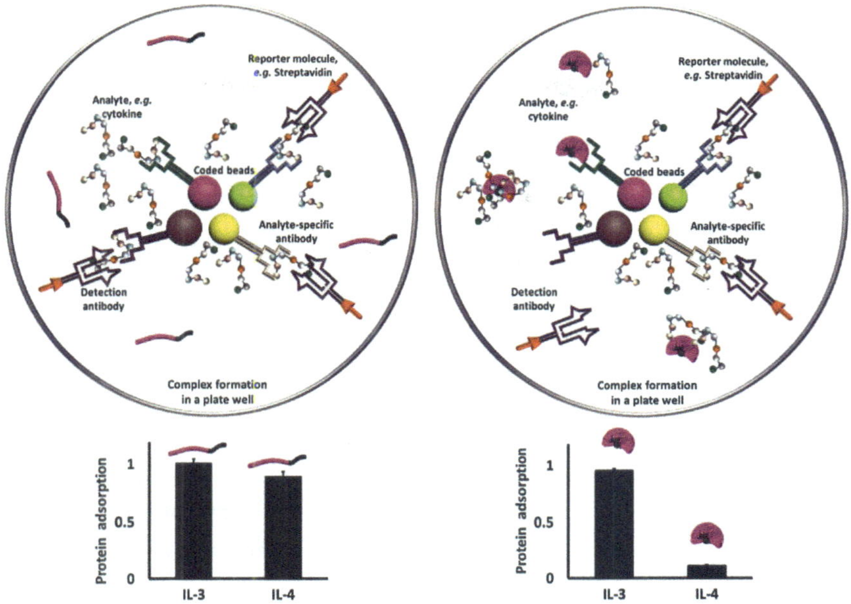

Figure 6.1 Schematic diagram that demonstrates the possible interference of nanomaterials with the multiplexing assay (right panel), as compared to nonassembled polymers (left panel). The two-column graphs represent the adsorption of IL-3 and IL-4 cytokines by poly(carboxybetaine)5k polymer and poly(carboxybetaine)5k-coated nanoparticles, which highlight the higher potential interference from nanoparticles, as compared to free polymers, and the difference in adsorption affinity across various cytokines. The values are presented as the ratio of concentrations of cytokines in the cytokine/nanoparticle mixture (500 μg/mL polymers or nanoparticles) to that in a solution that contains the same amount of the cytokines but without nanoparticles.

et al., 2009; Veranth et al., 2007). For a given cytokine, the extent of interaction with nanoparticles depends on the physicochemical characteristics of the nanoparticles, such as size, surface chemistry, hydrophobicity, and aspect ratio. Free polymers usually have a lower tendency to adsorb cytokines, as compared to assembled nanostructures, and adsorption affinity varies across various cytokines (Fig. 6.1) (Elsabahy et al., 2013).

Preassessment of the potential interactions between nanomaterials and cytokines, and, generally between biomarkers and tested materials, is crucial. This assessment can be carried out by incubating cytokines (standard solutions) with varying concentrations of nanomaterials, followed by measuring the concentrations of cytokines relative to their respective concentrations in the absence of the tested materials. Then, in the multiplexing experiments, nanomaterials shall be either used at concentrations that do not result in cytokine adsorption or interference with the complex formation, or the extent of cytokine adsorption should be accounted for in the analyses. Confirmatory tests can also be performed, for example, by measuring the intracellular and released proteins, and mRNA expression levels. However, this might be difficult and time consuming, as compared to the adsorption preassessment step, and still nanoparticles might be available to interact with RNA and proteins in the medium.

Nanomaterials have a tendency to adsorb proteins on their surfaces forming a loose network of proteins (i.e., protein corona) of various compositions (Kokkinopoulou et al., 2017). Adsorption of cytokines on nanomaterials during multiplexing assays would lead to underestimation of their expression levels. The preassessment step is of particular importance for studies that measure the dose-dependent effect of nanomaterials, as the adsorption of cytokines might increase upon increasing the concentrations of the tested nanoparticles. The same concept and precautions shall be taken into consideration for experiments that test the effect of micro- or nano-particles on the expression of various biomarkers (not only cytokines). The suggested preassessment strategy would allow for a better understanding of the immune response to the tested materials and will aid in the construction of pharmaceutical nanocarriers and medical devices of high safety profiles.

References

Dobrovolskaia, M. A., & McNeil, S. E. (2007). Immunological properties of engineered nanomaterials. *Nature Nanotechnology*, *2*(8), 469–478. Available from https://doi.org/10.1038/nnano.2007.223.

Elsabahy, M., Heo, G. S., Lim, S. M., Sun, G., & Wooley, K. L. (2015). Polymeric nanostructures for imaging and therapy. *Chemical Reviews*, *115*(19), 10967–11011. Available from https://doi.org/10.1021/acs.chemrev.5b00135.

Elsabahy, M., Li, A., Zhang, F., Sultan, D., Liu, Y., & Wooley, K. L. (2013). Differential immunotoxicities of poly(ethylene glycol)- vs. poly(carboxybetaine)-coated nanoparticles. *Journal of Controlled Release*, *172*(3), 641–652. Available from https://doi.org/10.1016/j.jconrel.2013.09.010.

Elsabahy, M., & Wooley, K. L. (2013). Cytokines as biomarkers of nanoparticle immunotoxicity. *Chemical Society Reviews*, *42*(12), 5552–5576. Available from https://doi.org/10.1039/c3cs60064e.

Elsabahy, M., & Wooley, K. L. (2015). Data mining as a guide for the construction of cross-linked nanoparticles with low immunotoxicity via control of polymer chemistry and supramolecular assembly. *Accounts of Chemical Research*, *48*(6), 1620–1630. Available from https://doi.org/10.1021/acs.accounts.5b00066.

Hunter, C. A., & Jones, S. A. (2015). IL-6 as a keystone cytokine in health and disease. *Nature Immunology*, *16*(5), 448–457. Available from https://doi.org/10.1038/ni.3153.

Hussain, S., Boland, S., Baeza-Squiban, A., Hamel, R., Thomassen, L. C. J., Martens, J. A., Billon-Galland, M. A., Fleury-Feith, J., Moisan, F., Pairon, J. C., & Marano, F. (2009). Oxidative stress and proinflammatory effects of carbon black and titanium dioxide nanoparticles: Role of particle surface area and internalized amount. *Toxicology*, *260*(1–3), 142–149. Available from https://doi.org/10.1016/j.tox.2009.04.001.

Jani, D., Allinson, J., Berisha, F., Cowan, K. J., Devanarayan, V., Gleason, C., Jeromin, A., Keller, S., Khan, M. U., Nowatzke, B., Rhyne, P., & Stephen, L. (2016). Recommendations for use and fit-for-purpose validation of biomarker multiplex ligand binding assays in drug development. *AAPS Journal*, *18*(1), 1–14. Available from https://doi.org/10.1208/s12248-015-9820-y.

Kocbach, A., Totlandsdal, A. I., Låg, M., Refsnes, M., & Schwarze, P. E. (2008). Differential binding of cytokines to environmentally relevant particles: A possible source for misinterpretation of in vitro results? *Toxicology Letters*, *176*(2), 131–137. Available from https://doi.org/10.1016/j.toxlet.2007.10.014.

Kokkinopoulou, M., Simon, J., Landfester, K., Mailänder, V., & Lieberwirth, I. (2017). Visualization of the protein corona: Towards a biomolecular understanding of nanoparticle-cell interactions. *Nanoscale*, *9*(25), 8858–8870. Available from https://doi.org/10.1039/c7nr02977b.

O'Shea, J. J., Ma, A., & Lipsky, P. (2002). Cytokines and autoimmunity. *Nature Reviews Immunology*, *2*(1), 37–45. Available from https://doi.org/10.1038/nri702.

Val, S., Hussain, S., Boland, S., Hamel, R., Baeza-Squiban, A., & Marano, F. (2009). Carbon black and titanium dioxide nanoparticles induce pro-inflammatory responses in bronchial epithelial cells: Need for multiparametric evaluation due to adsorption artifacts. *Inhalation Toxicology*, *21*(1), 115–122. Available from https://doi.org/10.1080/08958370902942533.

Veranth, J. M., Kaser, E. G., Veranth, M. M., Koch, M., & Yost, G. S. (2007). Cytokine responses of human lung cells (BEAS-2B) treated with micron-sized and nanoparticles of metal oxides compared to soil dusts. *Particle and Fibre Toxicology*, *4*.

CHAPTER 7

Data analysis and interpretation*

Mahmoud Elsabahy[1,2,3] and Karen L. Wooley[2]
[1]School of Biotechnology and Science Academy, Badr University in Cairo, Badr City, Cairo, Egypt
[2]Department of Chemistry, Laboratory for Synthetic-Biologic Interactions, Texas A&M University, College Station, TX, United States
[3]Misr University for Science and Technology, 6th of October City, Giza, Egypt

There are various therapeutic and diagnostic agents under development for several biomedical applications, with multiple approaches being applied to overcome intricate challenges toward their translation into clinically viable products (Arnold et al., 2017; Houdaihed et al., 2017; Leroux, 2017). Various biomarkers are currently being used for in vitro and in vivo preclinical and clinical testing during the development of drugs and biotechnology-based products and for diagnosis and monitoring of disease treatment, progression, and recurrence (Dobrovolskaia, 2015; Elsabahy & Wooley, 2013, 2018; Elsabahy, Li, et al., 2013; Elsabahy, Shrestha, et al., 2013; Elsabahy, Zhang, et al., 2013; Hong & Dobrovolskaia, 2019; Ilinskaya & Dobrovolskaia, 2016; Shrestha et al., 2012). Multiplexing technologies have reduced the required analysis times and sample sizes and have allowed for simultaneous analyses of up to hundreds of biomarkers in a few microliter sample volumes, with high sensitivity and accuracy (Elsabahy et al., 2019). Herein, we describe a data mining strategy that yields four descriptive values for each tested material, for quantitative assessment of multiple biomarkers, which facilitates direct comparative analyses across materials platforms.

Significant advancement in multiple analyte profiling has been achieved thanks to technological breakthroughs in polychromatic flow cytometry and multiplexing techniques that are capable of generating intensive amounts of data. Although the problem of comparing the levels of hundreds of biomarkers across different sets of materials is well recognized, little has been done toward intensive data management and interpretation. Comparing data across various laboratories is tedious and currently impractical, due to variations in the types of assays, experimental

* Adapted with permission from Elsabahy, M., Wooley, K. L., Hendricksen, A., & Oh, K. (2021). Multiple analyte profiling (MAP) index as a powerful diagnostic and therapeutic monitoring tool. *Methods, 190*, 26–32. https://doi.org/10.1016/j.ymeth.2020.03.006.

Immunomodulatory Effects of Nanomaterials
DOI: https://doi.org/10.1016/B978-0-323-90604-3.00002-4

setups, and conditions, in particular, when up to 500 markers can be currently assessed in one sample for one particular type of biomaterials. Unfortunately, this lack of adequate data mining and management techniques limits the ability of scientists to optimally use the generated data and necessitates the development of analytical tools that can provide descriptive values for the tested materials that are sufficiently simple for nonexperts to use (e.g., the use of IC_{50} and LD_{50} for in vitro and in vivo toxicity testing, respectively) (Chaussabel et al., 2009).

Data can be mined in a particular way to provide a convenient and robust algorithm to evaluate the expression of several biomarkers via the use of the multiple analyte profiling (MAP) index (Fig. 7.1), as described in Eq. (7.1):

$$MAP\ index = \sum_{i=1}^{n} \frac{Biomarker_i}{Control} \tag{7.1}$$

where $Biomarker_i$ and *Control* are the expression levels of a particular (i) biomarker (e.g., cytokine) induced by the tested material or expressed in a particular setup (e.g., disease or pathological condition), and the control, respectively.

Controls should be carefully included in the experiments, which could be either untreated cells or plasma/serum from animals injected with saline, for in vitro and in vivo assays, respectively. Worth mentioning is

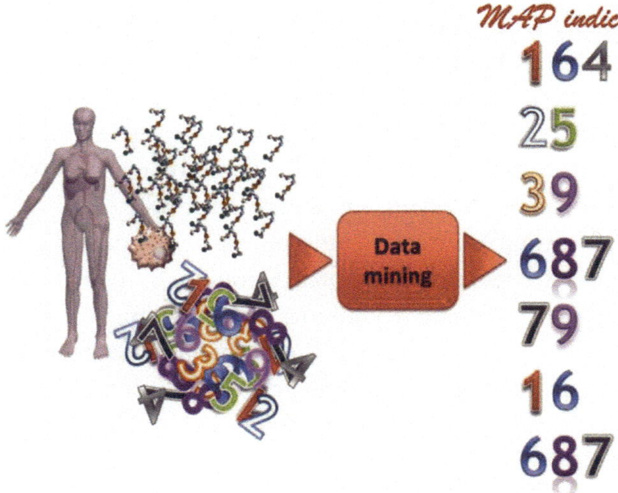

Figure 7.1 Data mined using the MAP index-based algorithm. It can be used for easier data mining and interpretation, and fair comparisons between data from various sources.

that these indices differ from in vitro to in vivo experiments, which might be due to the different environment (simple tissue culture medium versus complex blood components and plasma proteins) and dilution of biomarkers with significantly larger blood volume in vivo. Controls could be also represented by the biomarkers expression in healthy subjects compared to the same biomarkers expression in patients. Furthermore, subjects before treatment or vaccination may be utilized as controls to assess the effects of treatment or vaccination, respectively, in a particular disease model. There could be different terminology assignments for the calculated index. Initially, we had developed this technique to address challenges in assessing the immunotoxic effects within and across materials. We, therefore, apply the term immunotoxicity index, which can be used to assess the immunotoxic effect of the tested materials via measuring the expression levels of proinflammatory cytokines. This immunotoxicity index provides a single descriptive value for each nanoparticle type (under specified and defined experimental conditions), to be used as a valuable guide for the clinical development of pharmaceuticals and medical devices. Using this strategy, hundreds of numbers and figures (when the data are presented in individual figures for each cytokine) could be converted into a few numerical values and illustrative figures that are in agreement with the corresponding published data. This process allows for quantitative comparisons to be made between different sets of tested materials (Elsabahy & Wooley, 2015).

In the refined algorithm presented here, there are four types of MAP indices. Cumulative and absolute indices include or exclude the statistically insignificant expression of biomarkers (as compared to the control), respectively. Hence, in the absolute index, only biomarkers with significantly ($P < .05$, or as set by the analyst) different expressions as compared to the control are included. Furthermore, cumulative and absolute MAP indices can be utilized to account for overexpression and downregulation of biomarkers. Hence, the four MAP indices (i.e., cumulative and absolute indices for up- and downregulations of biomarkers) provide comprehensive information on the change of the biomarker map in response to treatment with a particular pharmaceutical agent or medical device or for diagnostic and therapeutic monitoring applications. The values of the indices might be utilized to compare between various samples across the study. However, for universal use and to allow other users to perform comparison studies and for the generation of a biomarker data bank, some essential parameters shall be defined because they directly influence the magnitude of the indices, such as the following:

1. In vitro and in vivo conditions: Incubation time, sampling time, cell type, animal/human disease status, etc.
2. Concentration of the tested materials.
3. Type: Cumulative or absolute and overexpression or downregulation.
4. Number and type of biomarkers used for calculation.
5. Statistical analysis probability value (*P* value).

Mining data using the suggested strategy would allow for a better understanding of disease progression, the biological (e.g., immune) response to the tested materials, fair comparisons between data from various sources, and is expected to generate useful guidelines for the construction of pharmaceutical carriers and medical devices of high safety profiles. The strategy has been applied to data available in the literature from our group and others, and impressive outcomes have been attained. Herein, we present examples for a description of the first application of the new algorithm as a powerful diagnostic and therapeutic monitoring tool in the management of breast cancer, as a disease model.

Breast cancer is the second most common cancer in American women and is the second leading cause of cancer death in women, with an increasing incidence rate in westernized countries, where early detection is crucial in lowering the mortality rate (Greenwood, 2019; Henriksen et al., 2019; Ma et al., 2019). Biomarkers are routinely measured for diagnosis of breast cancer as they have an effect on promoting or inhibiting the growth of breast cancer (Al-Hassan, 2013; Kim et al., 2009; Ławicki et al., 2013; Li et al., 2017). Various biomarkers have been measured to evaluate their prognostic values in breast cancer (Al-Hassan, 2013; Kim et al., 2009; Li et al., 2017). The advancement of multiplexing technologies, which allowed the simultaneous analyses of up to 500 biomarkers in a few microliter sample volumes, suffered from the side-by-side development of mathematical models and algorithms for digestion of the intensive data generated (Ma et al., 2019).

Multiplexing techniques have been utilized for the measurement of proinflammatory cytokines upon in vitro or in vivo treatment with nanomaterials of various structures and compositions. At that time, the only available strategy was to compare the levels of cytokines one by one, which was tedious and time consuming (Elsabahy, Li, et al., 2013; Elsabahy, Samarajeewa, et al., 2013; Elsabahy, Shrestha, et al., 2013; Elsabahy, Zhang, et al., 2013; Shrestha et al., 2012; Zhang et al., 2013).

Therefore we developed a simple mathematical equation to compare the ability of the nanomaterials to enhance the expression of cytokines via single descriptive values (i.e., the immunotoxicity index) (Elsabahy & Wooley, 2015). This technique could partially address challenges in assessing the immunotoxic effects within and across materials, where hundreds of numbers and figures could be transformed into few numerical values and illustrative figures that are in agreement with the corresponding published data (Elsabahy & Wooley, 2015).

In this chapter, we describe the use of a refined algorithm to evaluate the expression of several biomarkers via the use of the MAP index (Formula 7.1). Herein, we highlight the application of MAP indices as a diagnostic algorithm via analyzing data available in the literature. The literature data were selected randomly from articles that use various biomarkers for the diagnosis of breast cancer and report the mean or median values and the level of statistical significance (i.e., *P* value). The scope of some of these studies has been expanded beyond the utilization of biomarkers for diagnosis of breast cancer, to be exploited for the evaluation of the effect of treatment and vaccination on disease progression, and for differentiation between various subtypes or stages of breast cancer. We assessed the ability of the newly developed MAP indices to evaluate these different circumstances and the extent to which this concept could also be applied to select the most appropriate biomarker panel for a particular purpose (i.e., diagnostic, therapeutic monitoring, vaccination, disease categorization, etc.).

In one study, changes in the serum levels of three proinflammatory cytokines (IL-1α, IL-6, and TNF-α) were examined in breast cancer patients. In addition, the correlations between cancer progression and the expression of those biomarkers were investigated (Al-Hassan, 2013). Serum levels of the proinflammatory cytokines were higher in breast cancer patients as compared to the benign breast lesions group and the healthy control group. This increase was significantly associated with advanced stages of the disease. The values of the MAP indices are in complete agreement with the study outcomes. In addition, it is clearly seen how categorization of the breast cancer cases, according to stages, influenced the MAP index value (i.e., the MAP index significantly increased at higher stages [Fig. 7.2 and Table 7.1 (Al-Hassan, 2013)]. The low values of the cumulative MAP index (−) and absolute MAP index (−) (green and black squares, respectively, Fig. 7.2) indicate that there was no down-regulation, either significant or not, of the measured biomarkers in all

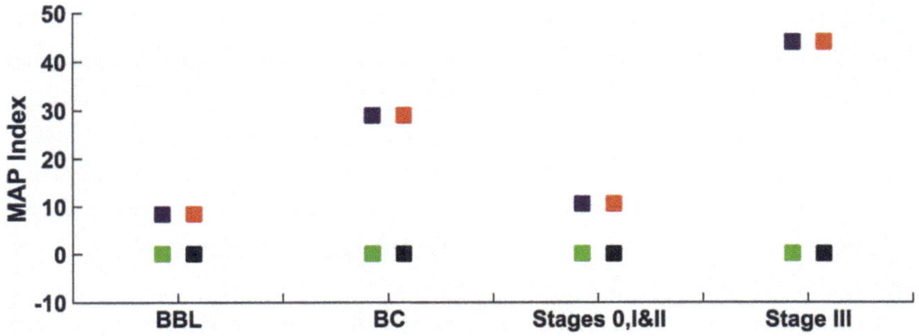

Figure 7.2 The MAP indices for the median serum levels of proinflammatory cytokines in BBL, BC, and healthy controls. Proinflammatory cytokines (IL-1α, IL-6, and TNF-α) in benign breast lesions group (BBL, $n = 12$), breast cancer patients (BC, $n = 45$), stages 0, I, and II patients ($n = 28$), and stage III patients ($n = 17$), as compared to the healthy control group ($n = 23$). The blue, green, red, and black squares refer to the cumulative MAP index (+), cumulative MAP index (−), absolute MAP index (+), and absolute MAP index (−), respectively.

Table 7.1 The MAP indices for the median serum levels of proinflammatory cytokines in breast cancer.

	BBL	BC cases	Stages 0, I, and II	Stage III
Cumulative MAP index (+)	8.4	28.9	10.5	43.9
Cumulative MAP index (−)	0	0	0	0
Absolute MAP index (+)	8.4	28.9	10.5	43.9
Absolute MAP index (−)	0	0	0	0

The MAP indices for the median serum levels of proinflammatory cytokines (IL-1α, IL-6, and TNF-α) in benign breast lesions group (BBL, $n = 12$), breast cancer patients (BC, $n = 45$), stages 0, I, and II patients ($n = 28$), and stage III patients ($n = 17$), as compared to the healthy control group ($n = 23$).

groups. On the contrary, blue and red squares refer to the cumulative MAP index (+) and absolute MAP index (+), respectively, and were clearly of greater values in the breast cancer patients as compared to the benign breast lesions group and the healthy control group, and these values increased in patients at higher stages (Stage III), as compared to lower stages of the disease (Stages 0, I, and II). It can be concluded that combining stages of breast cancer might not be useful and/or those biomarkers are more appropriate for the prediction of higher stages of the disease [see the blue and red squares of the BC group that have intermediate values (higher than that of the "Stages 0, I, and II" group and lower than the values of the "Stage III" group)]. The equal values of the cumulative and absolute indices [either (+) or (−)] in this study demonstrate that, when the expression of biomarkers changes, those changes were all statistically significant ($P < .05$).

In another study, plasma levels of several hematopoietic cytokines were measured in breast cancer patients, benign breast tumor patients, and healthy subjects (Ławicki et al., 2013). Plasma levels were higher in the breast cancer patients, as compared to the healthy control groups, and this increase was significant in patients at advanced stages of the disease. The values of the MAP indices are in complete agreement with the study findings (Fig. 7.3 and Table 7.2) (Ławicki et al., 2013). The application of MAP indices in both studies (Figs. 7.2 and 7.3) highlights that combining all stages in comparative studies may result in biased data analysis (Al-Hassan, 2013; Ławicki et al., 2013). Higher stages are associated with significantly higher expression of cytokines as compared to the control group and patients with a benign tumor, and thus those markers might be useful only for the diagnosis of patients at advanced stages of the disease. Those biomarkers may distinguish patients at different stages of breast cancer from healthy subjects, but only differentiate patients at advanced stages of the disease from patients with benign tumors. Data mining and analysis using the MAP indices provided detailed information on the expression

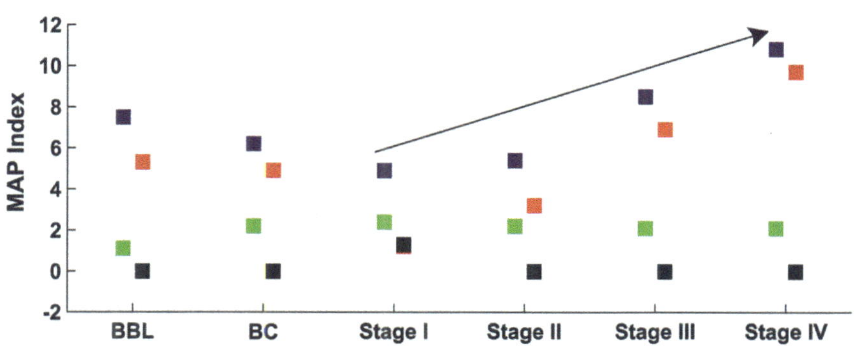

Figure 7.3 The MAP indices for the median plasma levels of IL-3, stem cell factor (SCF), granulocyte-macrophage colony-stimulating factor (GM-CSF), granulocyte colony-stimulating factor (G-CSF) and macrophage colony-stimulating factor (M-CSF), and the tumor marker carcinoma antigen 15−3 (CA 15−3) in the BBL ($n = 40$), BC patients ($n = 110$), and patients at stages I ($n = 25$), II ($n = 35$), III ($n = 25$) and IV ($n = 25$), as compared to the healthy control group ($n = 40$). The blue, green, red, and black squares refer to the cumulative MAP index (+), cumulative MAP index (−), absolute MAP index (+), and absolute MAP index (−), respectively. The arrow indicates the increase in the values of the cumulative MAP index (+) and absolute MAP index (+) for patients at higher stages of breast cancer.

Table 7.2 The MAP indices for the median plasma levels of IL-3, stem cell factor (SCF), granulocyte-macrophage colony-stimulating factor (GM-CSF), granulocyte colony-stimulating factor (G-CSF) and macrophage colony-stimulating factor (M-CSF), and the tumor marker carcinoma antigen 15−3 (CA 15−3).

	BBL	BC	Stage I	Stage II	Stage III	Stage IV
Cumulative MAP index (+)	7.5	6.2	4.9	5.4	8.5	10.8
Cumulative MAP index (−)	1.1	2.2	2.4	2.2	2.1	2.1
Absolute MAP index (+)	5.3	4.9	1.2	3.2	6.9	9.7
Absolute MAP index (−)	0	0	1.3	0	0	0

patterns of the biomarkers at various stages of the disease. It can be observed that there was slight downregulation in some biomarkers, but with no statistical significance from the healthy subjects [look at the absolute MAP index (−) values, the black squares]. Clearly, higher expression of the biomarkers was observed in patients with breast cancer, and these expression levels increased for patients at higher stages of the disease (blue and red squares). Although the MAP indices in Figs. 7.2 and 7.3 have different values, it can be clearly concluded that those biomarkers may distinguish patients at advanced stages of the disease from patients with benign tumors. The differences in values of the MAP indices in Figs. 7.2 and 7.3 were expected, due to the variations in the number and type of the measured biomarkers, in addition to differences in the other experimental conditions.

The MAP indices for the median plasma levels of these markers in BBL ($n = 40$), BC patients ($n = 110$), and patients at stages I ($n = 25$), II ($n = 35$), III ($n = 25$), and IV ($n = 25$), as compared to the healthy control group ($n = 40$).

Similar to the two previous studies, Lyon et al. compared the plasma levels of 17 selected cytokines in breast cancer patients to those in benign and healthy control groups. Significantly higher expression of the biomarkers was found in breast cancer patients (Lyon et al., 2011). The values of the MAP indices are in complete agreement with the study conclusions [Fig. 7.4 and Table 7.3 (Lyon et al., 2011)]. It is clearly demonstrated that both patients in the benign tumor and breast cancer groups can be distinguished from the healthy groups. Breast cancer patients can also be differentiated from patients with benign tumors. The advantage of utilizing MAP indices in data mining and analysis was more evident in this study, due to the higher number of the measured biomarkers (Henriksen et al., 2019),

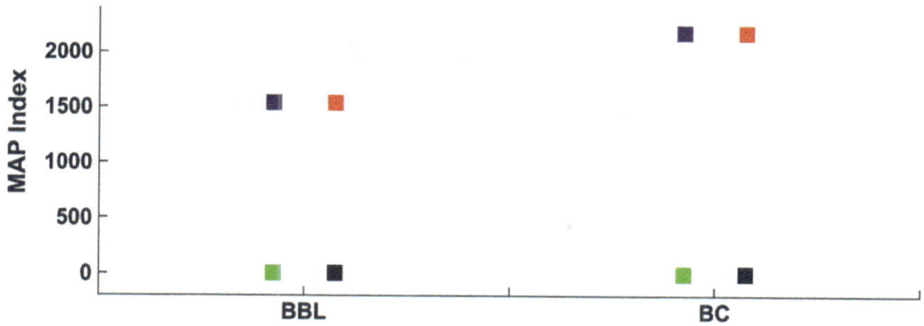

Figure 7.4 The MAP indices for the median plasma levels of 17 cytokines. Cytokines including IL-1β, IL-2, IL-4, IL-5, IL-6, IL-7, IL-8, IL-10, IL-12, IL-13, IL-17, granulocyte colony-stimulating factor (G-CSF), granulocyte-macrophage colony-stimulating factor (GM-CSF), interferon-γ (IFN-γ), monocyte chemotactic protein-1 (MCP-1), macrophage inflammatory protein-1β (MIP-1β), and tumor necrosis factor-α (TNF-α) in the BBL patients ($n = 24$) and BC patients ($n = 33$), as compared to the healthy control group ($n = 33$). The blue, green, red, and black squares refer to the cumulative MAP index (+), cumulative MAP index (−), absolute MAP index (+), and absolute MAP index (−), respectively.

Table 7.3 The MAP indices for the median plasma levels of 17 cytokines in BBL.

	BBL	BC
Cumulative MAP index (+)	1539.9	2186.9
Cumulative MAP index (−)	4.3	0
Absolute MAP index (+)	1539.9	2185.9
Absolute MAP index (−)	3.3	0

compared to the two previous examples (3 and 6 biomarkers in Figs. 7.2 and 7.3, respectively). A higher number of biomarkers usually increases the complexity during the management of the generated data, whereas it does not affect the analysis using the newly developed algorithm that generates only four descriptive values for each group. Interestingly, the MAP indices might be also applied to patient by patient rather than the median of each group to provide more detailed information on each patient. Unfortunately, we had access to the median values of the various groups, but data for each individual patient were not available.

The MAP indices for the median plasma levels of 17 cytokines, IL-1β, IL-2, IL-4, IL-5, IL-6, IL-7, IL-8, IL-10, IL-12, IL-13, IL-17, granulocyte colony-stimulating factor (G-CSF), granulocyte-macrophage colony-stimulating factor (GM-CSF), interferon-γ (IFN-γ), monocyte chemotactic protein-1 (MCP-1), macrophage inflammatory protein-1β (MIP-1β), and tumor necrosis factor-α (TNF-α) in the BBL patients ($n = 24$) and BC patients ($n = 33$), as compared to the healthy control group ($n = 33$).

The use of the MAP index was then examined in a study that involved a higher number of analytes. The aim of this study was to examine the potential use of 35 analytes as a profiling signature for primary nonmetastatic breast cancer for diagnostic purposes (Kim et al., 2009). Serum levels of the biomarkers were higher in breast cancer patients as compared to the healthy control group (98 women vs 96 healthy women). Interestingly, the authors had grouped the biomarkers to select the most appropriate diagnostic group. The values of the MAP indices are in complete agreement with the study conclusions [Fig. 7.5 and Table 7.4 (Kim et al., 2009)]. In addition, the MAP indices could be generated for each group of biomarkers, as in the study, to aid in efficient and rapid

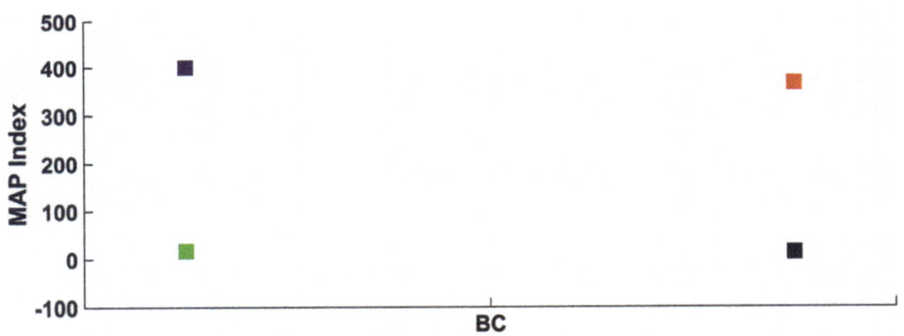

Figure 7.5 The MAP indices for the grouped biomarkers (35 analytes) in the BC. The MAP indices for the grouped biomarkers (35 analytes) in the BC patients ($n = 98$), as compared to the healthy control group ($n = 96$). The blue, green, red, and black squares refer to the cumulative MAP index (+), cumulative MAP index (−), absolute MAP index (+), and absolute MAP index (−), respectively. The arrow refers to the superimposed absolute MAP indices (+) and (−).

Table 7.4 The MAP indices for the mean serum levels of 35 analytes in BC.

	BC
Cumulative MAP index (+)	400.1
Cumulative MAP index (−)	17.5
Absolute MAP index (+)	363.9
Absolute MAP index (−)	13.4

The MAP indices for the mean serum levels of 35 analytes in the BC patients ($n = 98$), as compared to the healthy control group ($n = 96$).

screening of biomarkers and to select the most suitable diagnostic panel for future use in the diagnosis of breast cancer [Fig. 7.6 and Table 7.5 (Kim et al., 2009)]. For instance, it is clear from the absolute MAP index (+) value that the immune/inflammation group of biomarkers (i.e., soluble CD40 ligand (sCD40L), β2-microglobulin and myeloperoxidase) is the most informative diagnostic group that can be exploited in the diagnosis of breast cancer, in comparison to the other groups that include the other 32 measured analytes. Among the immune/inflammation group of biomarkers, serum concentrations of sCD40L showed the most significant increase in breast cancer patients compared to normal subjects [Tables 7.6 and 7.7 (Kim et al., 2009)]. There is an association between elevated plasma levels of sCD40L and tumor progression, probably due to the enhancement of the procoagulant activity of tumor cells through upregulation of tissue factor expression, thus promoting angiogenesis and platelet activation (Kim et al., 2009).

In a comprehensive study, serum levels of 19 cytokine profiles in breast cancer patients, healthy controls, node-positive patients, node-negative patients, and pre- and postvaccinated patients (patients vaccinated with HER2/*neu* E75 peptide vaccine), were examined (Dehqanzada et al., 2007). The proinflammatory state in the cancer patients increased as compared to normal healthy donors (i.e., higher expression of cytokines). A more pronounced proinflammatory state was also found in the node-negative patients compared to the node-positive patients. Furthermore, vaccination induced a more evident proinflammatory state. The values of

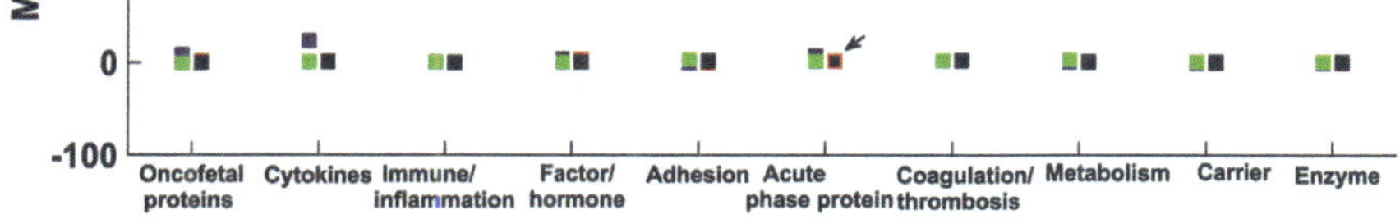

Figure 7.6 MAP indices for the mean serum levels of 35 analytes in BC. The MAP indices for the mean serum levels of 35 analytes in the BC patients ($n = 98$), as compared to the healthy control group ($n = 96$). The blue, green, red, and black squares refer to the cumulative MAP index (+), cumulative MAP index (−), absolute MAP index (+), and absolute MAP index (−), respectively.

Table 7.5 The MAP indices for the grouped biomarkers (35 analytes) in BC.

	Cumulative MAP index (+)	Cumulative MAP index (−)	Absolute MAP index (+)	Absolute MAP index (−)
Oncofetal protein Alpha-fetoprotein (AFP) Carcinoembryonic antigen (CEA) Cancer antigen 125 (CA125) Cancer antigen 19−9 (CA19−9) Prostate-specific antigen (PSA)	9.1	0	2.4	0
Cytokine IL-1β IL-1 receptor α IL-6 IL-8 Monocyte chemotactic protein-1 Monocyte inflammatory protein-1α	24.3	1.0	1.7	1.0
Immune/Inflammation Soluble CD40 ligand β2-microglobulin Myeloperoxidase	350.3	1.0	348.9	0
Factor/hormone Epidermal growth factor (EGF) Adiponectin	4.2	1.1	4.2	1.1
Adhesion Vitronectin Soluble vascular cell adhesion molecule-1 Soluble intercellular cell adhesion molecule-1	0	3.4	0	2.3
Acute phase protein Alpha-1-antitrypin Alpha-2 macroglobulin C-reactive protein D-dimer Haptoglobin α Serum amyloid A Transthyretin	7.9	2.3	2.3	2.3

(*Continued*)

Table 7.5 (Continued)

	Cumulative MAP index (+)	Cumulative MAP index (−)	Absolute MAP index (+)	Absolute MAP index (−)
Coagulation/thrombosis Hemoglobin High-molecular-weight kininogen Plasminogen activator inhibitor-1	3.0	2.9	3.0	2.9
Metabolism Apolipoprotein A1 Pro-apolipoprotein A1 Apolipoprotein A4 Apolipoprotein H	1.2	3.5	1.2	1.4
Carrier Vitamin D-binding protein	0	1.1	0	1.1
Enzyme Cathepsin B	0	1.1	0	1.1

The MAP indices for the grouped biomarkers (35 analytes) in the BC patients ($n = 98$), as compared to the healthy control group ($n = 96$).

Table 7.6 The MAP indices for the immune/inflammation individual biomarkers.

Biomarker	Cumulative MAP index (+)	Cumulative MAP index (−)	Absolute MAP index (+)	Absolute MAP index (−)
Soluble CD40 ligand	348.9	0	348.9	0
β2-microglobulin	0	1.0	0	0
Myeloperoxidase	1.3	0	0	0

The MAP indices for the median serum levels of 19 selected cytokines in the BC patients ($n = 22$), as compared to the healthy control group ($n = 13$), for the node-negative patients ($n = 24$) as compared to the node-positive patients ($n = 12$), and for the postvaccinated patients ($n = 34$) as compared to the patients before vaccination ($n = 34$). The blue, green, red, and black squares refer to the cumulative MAP index (+), cumulative MAP index (−), absolute MAP index (+), and absolute MAP index (−), respectively.

the MAP indices are in complete agreement with the findings from the study that the expression of selected cytokines had increased in breast cancer patients versus normal subjects, due to the ongoing or previous endogenous anticancer immune response [Fig. 7.7 (Anber et al., 2016) and Table 7.8 (Dehqanzada et al., 2007)]. Furthermore, the MAP

Table 7.7 The expression levels of the immune/inflammation individual biomarkers in BC.

Biomarker	Normal ($n = 96$)	BC ($n = 98$)	*P* value
Soluble CD40 ligand (pg/mL)	32.17	11,226.31	<.001
β2-microglobulin (ng/mL)	720.68	692.36	.125
Myeloperoxidase (pg/mL)	1,12,079.27	1,46,459.9	.233

The expression levels of the immune/inflammation individual biomarkers (soluble CD40 ligand, β2-microglobulin, and myeloperoxidase) in the BC patients ($n = 98$), as compared to the healthy control group ($n = 96$).

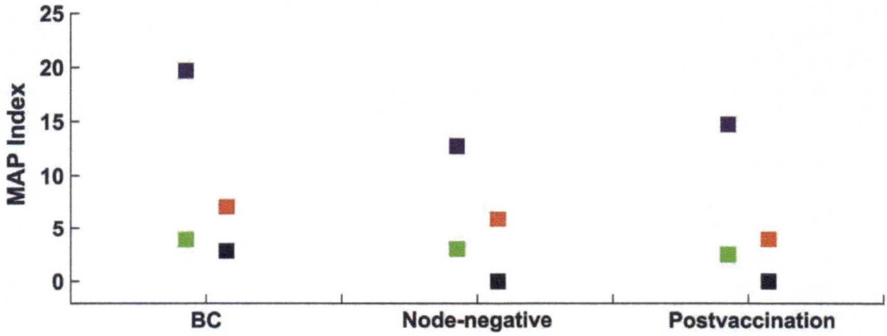

Figure 7.7 The MAP indices for the median serum levels of 19 selected cytokines in the BC. The MAP indices for the median serum levels of 19 selected cytokines in the BC patients ($n = 22$), as compared to the healthy control group ($n = 13$), for the node-negative patients ($n = 24$) as compared to the node-positive patients ($n = 12$), and for the postvaccinated patients ($n = 34$) as compared to the patients before vaccination ($n = 34$). The blue, green, red, and black squares refer to the cumulative MAP index (+), cumulative MAP index (−), absolute MAP index (+), and absolute MAP index (−), respectively.

Table 7.8 The MAP indices for the median serum levels of 19 selected cytokines in BC.

	BC	Node-negative	Postvaccination
Cumulative MAP index (+)	**19.7**	12.7	14.7
Cumulative MAP index (−)	3.9	3.0	2.5
Absolute MAP index (+)	7.1	5.9	3.9
Absolute MAP index (−)	2.8	0	0

The MAP indices for the median serum levels of 19 selected cytokines in the BC patients ($n = 22$) as compared to the healthy control group ($n = 13$), for the node-negative patients ($n = 24$) as compared to the node-positive patients ($n = 12$), and for the postvaccinated patients ($n = 34$) as compared to the patients before vaccination ($n = 34$).

indices were useful to provide descriptive values to differentiate between the two subtypes of breast cancer patients (i.e., node-negative vs node-positive) and to evaluate the effect of vaccination on the proinflammatory status of the patients. The MAP index (−) values indicate that downregulation of the measured biomarkers was of least importance. In contrast, overexpression of the measured biomarkers was clearly evident. However, it should be noted that the values for the breast cancer patients, node-negative, and postvaccinated groups of Fig. 7.7, should not be compared against each other, but rather versus the healthy control group, node-positive patients, and patients before vaccination, respectively.

A characteristic pattern was found in one more study that evaluated the levels of 274 biomarkers in breast cancer patients as compared to the control healthy group (Li et al., 2017). Among the initially tested 274 biomarkers, the serum levels of IL-8, MIP-1α, MIP-1β, MMP-8, Resistin, Follistatin-related gene protein (FLRG), and breast cancer attractor metagenes (BCAM) were significantly higher in breast cancer patients, latency associated peptide (LAP) and TSH-β levels were significantly lower, as compared to the healthy subjects. The values of the MAP indices are in complete agreement with the conclusions from the study [Fig. 7.8 and Table 7.9 (Li et al., 2017)]. From the values of the MAP indices, it is clear that they can be utilized for evaluating

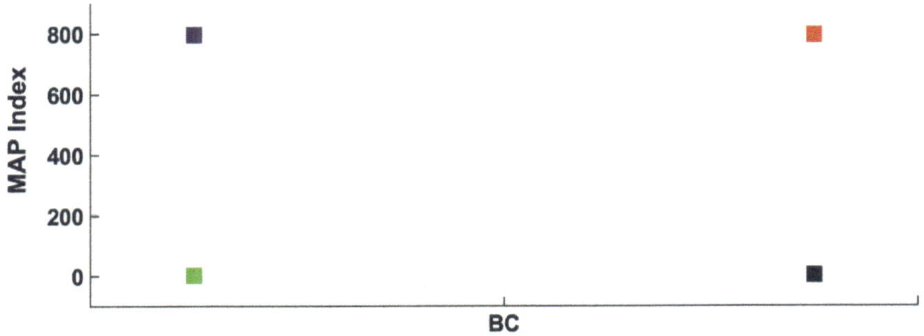

Figure 7.8 The MAP indices for the mean serum levels of nine selected biomarkers in BC. The MAP indices for the mean serum levels of nine selected biomarkers (out of 274 biomarkers) in the BC patients ($n = 11$), as compared to the healthy control group ($n = 10$). The blue, green, red, and black squares refer to the cumulative MAP index (+), cumulative MAP index (−), absolute MAP index (+), and absolute MAP index (−), respectively.

Table 7.9 The MAP indices for the mean serum levels of nine selected biomarkers in BC.

	BC
Cumulative MAP index (+)	**796.9**
Cumulative MAP index (−)	2.8
Absolute MAP index (+)	796.9
Absolute MAP index (−)	2.8

The MAP indices for the mean serum levels of nine selected biomarkers (out of 274 biomarkers) in the BC patients ($n = 11$), as compared to the healthy control group ($n = 10$).

both upregulation and downregulation of biomarkers expression. Few biomarkers were significantly downregulated [absolute MAP index (−) = 2.8], whereas most were significantly upregulated [absolute MAP index (+) = 796.9]. Based on this study, for future use, it might be more appropriate to utilize the upregulated panel (i.e., IL-8, MIP-1α, MIP-1β, MMP-8, Resistin, FLRG, and BCAM) versus the downregulated panel (i.e., LAP and TSH-β), as the absolute MAP index (+) value of the upregulated panel is much higher than the absolute MAP index (−) of the downregulated one (796.9 vs 2.8).

The effect of treatment of breast cancer on the expression of cytokines was examined in one study via measurement of the serum levels of seven cytokines in breast cancer patients versus the healthy controls (Anber et al., 2016). There was a significant increase in inflammatory cytokines in breast cancer patients before treatment as compared to the controls. No significant differences were observed between the healthy controls and the breast cancer patients who were under treatment. Significantly higher expressions of the measured cytokines were demonstrated for the breast cancer patients as compared to the patients under treatment, either when compared against the same cases before and under treatment, or when the under-treatment group was compared against the total patients group. The values of the MAP indices are in complete agreement with the outcomes of the study, and thus they can be utilized to evaluate and monitor the effect of treatment on breast cancer progression [Fig. 7.9 and Table 7.10 (Anber et al., 2016)]. Superimposed absolute MAP indices (+) and (−) at zero value (arrow in Fig. 7.9 for comparison of the under-treatment group against the healthy control) indicate that there were no statistically significant differences (upregulation or downregulation) between the measured biomarkers in the two groups.

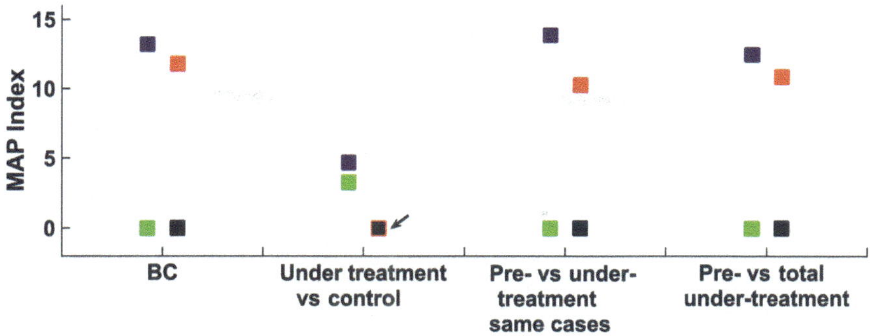

Figure 7.9 The MAP indices for the mean serum levels of seven cytokines in the BC. The MAP indices for the mean serum levels of seven cytokines in the BC patients ($n = 32$) as compared to the healthy control group ($n = 10$), patients under-treatment ($n = 36$) versus control ($n = 10$), pretreatment group ($n = 10$) versus the under-treatment group ($n = 10$) for the same cases, and pretreatment group ($n = 32$) versus the total under-treatment group ($n = 36$). The blue, green, red, and black squares refer to the cumulative MAP index (+), cumulative MAP index (−), absolute MAP index (+), and absolute MAP index (−), respectively. The arrow refers to the superimposed absolute MAP indices (+) and (−) at zero value.

Table 7.10 The MAP indices for the mean serum levels of seven cytokines in BC.

	BC	Under treatment versus control	Pre- versus under-treatment same cases	Pre- versus total under-treatment
Cumulative MAP index (+)	c	4.7	13.9	12.5
Cumulative MAP index (−)	0	3.3	0	0
Absolute MAP index (+)	11.8	0	10.3	10.9
Absolute MAP index (−)	0	0	0	0

The MAP indices for the mean serum levels of seven cytokines in the BC patients ($n = 32$) as compared to the healthy control group ($n = 10$), patients under-treatment ($n = 36$) versus control ($n = 10$), pretreatment group ($n = 10$) versus the under-treatment group ($n = 10$) for the same cases, and pretreatment group ($n = 32$) versus the total under-treatment group ($n = 36$).

7.1 Discussion

Breast cancer is the second most common cancer in American women and is the second leading cause of cancer death in women. Biomarkers have a great potential in minimally invasive detection of breast cancer, monitoring and assessment of therapy, and differentiation of subtypes, which is critical for the selection of the appropriate therapeutic regimen. Multiplexing technologies allow the simultaneous analyses of up to 500 biomarkers in a few microliter sample volumes. There are several experimental and technical challenges toward the use of multiplexing techniques that have been recently reviewed by our group (Elsabahy & Wooley, 2018; Elsabahy et al., 2019), and others (Jani et al., 2016). In addition, mathematical models and algorithms for the digestion of the intensive generated data are crucial for the optimal utilization of the assays and analysis of the data.

Comparing the levels of biomarkers one by one is tedious and time consuming. We have developed a simple mathematical equation to compare the ability of the nanomaterials to induce the expression of cytokines via single descriptive values (i.e., the immunotoxicity index) (Elsabahy & Wooley, 2015). Herein, we expanded its use to a more comprehensive algorithm to evaluate the expression of several biomarkers via the use of the MAP index [Formula (7.1)]. An example of the potential application of the new algorithm is being illustrated for breast cancer, as a disease model. MAP indices were calculated to provide information on breast cancer diagnosis, and evaluation of the effect of treatment and vaccination on the disease progression and for differentiation between various subtypes or stages of breast cancer. Furthermore, the use of the MAP indices to aid in the selection of the most appropriate biomarker panel for a particular purpose is illustrated.

There are four descriptive MAP indices for each group. The blue, green, red, and black squares of the figures (Figs. 7.2–7.9) refer to the cumulative MAP index (+), cumulative MAP index (−), absolute MAP index (+), and absolute MAP index (−), respectively. The values of the MAP indices for the included studies are demonstrated (Tables 7.1–7.10).

Generally, serum levels of the proinflammatory cytokines and other measured biomarkers were higher in breast cancer patients as compared to the benign breast lesions group and the healthy control group. This increase was significantly associated with advanced stages of the disease. The MAP indices could be generated for each panel of biomarker groups to aid in the selection of the most suitable panel for diagnostic purposes. Biomarker panels in Figs. 7.2 and 7.4 are more appropriate selection compared to the panel in Fig. 7.3, as can be seen from the differences in the MAP indices for the breast cancer patients versus the patients diagnosed with benign tumors (Figs. 7.2–7.4). Categorization of the breast cancer cases into stages influenced the MAP index value (i.e., the MAP index significantly increased at higher stages). Overexpression was more evident than the downregulation of the tested biomarkers. Biomarkers were more appropriate for the prediction of higher stages of the disease, whereas combining all stages in comparative studies may result in biased data interpretation. Differences in values of the MAP indices should be expected, due to variations in the number and type of the measured biomarkers, in addition to the differences in the other experimental conditions.

A higher number of biomarkers usually increases the complexity of traditional analytical methods, whereas it does not affect the analysis using the newly developed algorithm. The advantage of utilizing MAP indices in data mining and analysis is more evident in studies that involve high numbers (e.g., hundreds, thousands, etc.) of biomarkers. The MAP indices might be also applied to patient by patient rather than for the median of a group to provide a more detailed profiling of each patient.

MAP indices of the analyzed data were consistent and in agreement with the conclusions from each cited study, signifying their potential as a powerful tool for biomarkers data mining and analysis, for monitoring and diagnosis of various diseases, and for aid in the selection of the most appropriate biomarkers panels for a particular purpose. Worth mentioning is that the time required for extracting the MAP indices from the data set can range from a few hours manually to a few minutes using available software (e.g., MATLAB, MathWorks, Inc., Natick, MA).

7.2 Method

Experimental design: Experiments vary greatly depending on the purpose of the study, and whether experiments are designed to examine the biological or immunotoxic effects of biomaterials and medical devices, or being utilized to diagnose a disease, or to assess the effect of treatment or vaccination on disease progression. However, for comparison against other groups, all experimental conditions shall be fixed. For instance, for the detection of breast cancer in patients in comparison to data reported in the literature, the same types and number of the measured biomarkers shall be used, and all other experimental variables should be considered. Even if comparison against data available in the literature is not of concern, to assess the effect of treatment or vaccination on breast cancer progression, the same biomarkers shall be measured before and after treatment or vaccination. MAP indices values are directly correlated to the number of measured biomarkers and cannot be used to compare between two groups (e.g., breast cancer patients vs healthy subjects) unless the same types and numbers of the biomarkers are measured.

Data extraction: Either mean or median value should be calculated for a particular biomarker expression in each group. Statistical analysis probability value (*P* value) must be determined. Then, biomarkers should be categorized into two groups: one group that includes biomarkers that have higher expression levels (Table 7.11) and another group that involves biomarkers of lower expression levels (Table 7.12), as compared to the control or the group against which a comparison is made. Herein, an example is being presented for data illustrated in Fig. 7.8.

MAP indices: MAP indices shall be then calculated based on Formula (7.1):

There are four types of the estimated index, namely, cumulative and absolute MAP (+) and (−) indices, which include (i.e., cumulative) or exclude (i.e., absolute) the statistically insignificant overexpression [i.e., (+)] or downregulation [i.e., (−)] of biomarkers, as compared to the

Table 7.11 Overexpression of biomarkers in breast cancer.

Biomarker	Overexpression		
	Normal ($n = 10$)	Breast cancer ($n = 11$)	*P* value
MIP-1	7.591	5598.506	.000
IL-8	172.922	6081.530	.000
MIP-1β	572.697	7200.901	.000
Resistin	156.018	511.794	.001
FLRG	275.829	1056.580	.002
MMP-8	2285.479	6084.275	.001
BCAM	149.430	290.721	.001

Overexpression of biomarkers in breast cancer patients as compared to normal subjects (data presented in Fig. 7.8).

Table 7.12 Downregulation of biomarkers in breast cancer.

Biomarker	Downregulation		
	Normal ($n = 10$)	Breast cancer ($n = 11$)	*P* value
LAP	3160.995	2517.709	.045
TSH-β	493.926	305.149	.000

Downregulation of biomarkers in breast cancer patients as compared to normal subjects (data presented in Fig. 7.8).

Table 7.13 Normalized overexpression of biomarkers in breast cancer patients as compared to normal subjects (data presented in Fig. 7.8).

Biomarker	Overexpression in breast cancer
MIP-1α	737.519
IL-8	35.169
MIP-1β	12.574
Resistin	3.280
FLRG	3.831
MMP-8	2.662
BCAM	1.946
Cumulative MAP index (+)	796.981
Absolute MAP index (+)	796.981

The cumulative and absolute MAP indices (+) values are the summation of the values of the normalized overexpression. Cumulative and absolute indices are equal because overexpression was statistically significant for the seven biomarkers.

Table 7.14 Normalized downregulation of biomarkers in breast cancer patients as compared to normal subjects (data presented in Fig. 7.8).

Biomarker	Downregulation in breast cancer
LAP	1.256
TSH-β	1.619
Cumulative MAP index (−)	2.875
Absolute MAP index (−)	2.875

Normalized downregulation of biomarkers in breast cancer patients as compared to normal subjects (data presented in Fig. 7.8). The cumulative and absolute MAP indices (−) values are the summation of the values of the normalized downregulation. Cumulative and absolute indices are equal because downregulation was statistically significant for the two biomarkers.

control. Examples of the calculations of the four indices are provided in Tables 7.13 and 7.14.

Data interpretation: After calculation of the four descriptive MAP indices for each group (Tables 7.13 and 7.14), interpretation of the data should be straightforward. Furthermore, illustrative figures [Fig. 7.10 (Li et al., 2017)] are extremely useful to understand the change in the biomarkers map for a particular setup. Herein, several hints are provided as a guideline for data interpretation:

1. Low values of cumulative or absolute (+) or (−) indices indicate that overexpression or downregulation is of least importance, respectively.
2. High differences in values between cumulative and absolute MAP indices demonstrate that the differences in expression of the

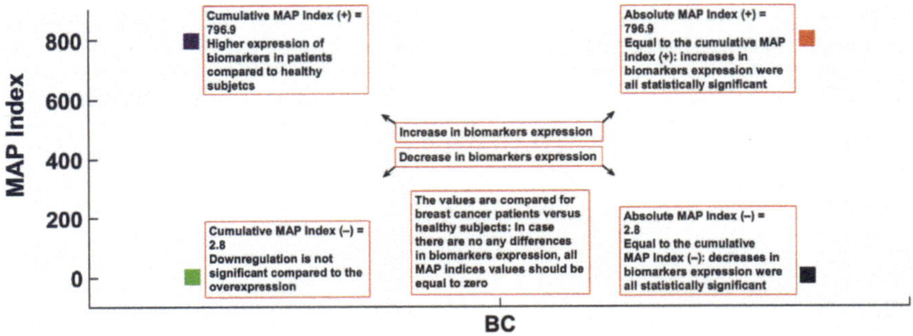

Figure 7.10 Illustration of the interpretation of the MAP indices for the mean serum levels of nine selected biomarkers in the breast cancer BC. The MAP indices calculated for the cytokines in Tables 7.13 and 7.14 are in breast cancer (BC) patients, as compared to the healthy control group.

biomarkers are not statistically significant for several of the measured biomarkers. In contrast, absolute and cumulative MAP indices will have the same values if variations in biomarkers expression are all statistically significant.

3. Superimposed absolute MAP indices (+) and (−) at zero value indicate that there are no statistically significant differences between the measured biomarkers in the two groups in comparison.
4. Absolute MAP indices could be only equal or less than the cumulative MAP indices.

References

Al-Hassan, A. A. (2013). Prognostic value of proinflammatory cytokines in breast cancer. *Journal of Biomolecular Research & Therapeutics*. Available from https://doi.org/10.4172/2167-7956.1000104.

Anber, N., EL-Sebaie, A. H., Mousa, S. A., & Elbaz, O. (2016). Expression of some inflammatory biomarkers in patients with breast cancer. *International Journal of Health Science Research*, *6*, 172−181.

Arnold, A. E., Czupiel, P., & Shoichet, M. (2017). Engineered polymeric nanoparticles to guide the cellular internalization and trafficking of small interfering ribonucleic acids. *Journal of Controlled Release*, *259*, 3−15. Available from https://doi.org/10.1016/j.jconrel.2017.02.019.

Chaussabel, D., Ueno, H., Banchereau, J., & Quinn, C. (2009). Data management: It starts at the bench. *Nature Immunology*, *10*(12), 1225−1227. Available from https://doi.org/10.1038/ni1209-1225.

Dehqanzada, Z. A., Storrer, C. E., Hueman, M. T., Foley, R. J., Harris, K. A., Jama, Y. H., Shriver, C. D., Ponniah, S., & Peoples, G. E. (2007). Assessing serum cytokine profiles in breast cancer patients receiving a HER2/neu vaccine using Luminex® technology. *Oncology Reports*, *17*(3), 687−694. Available from https://doi.org/10.3892/or.17.3.687.

Dobrovolskaia, M. A. (2015). Pre-clinical immunotoxicity studies of nanotechnology-formulated drugs: Challenges, considerations and strategy. *Journal of Controlled Release, 220*, 571–583. Available from https://doi.org/10.1016/j.jconrel.2015.08.056.

Elsabahy, M., & Wooley, K. L. (2013). Cytokines as biomarkers of nanoparticle immunotoxicity. *Chemical Society Reviews, 42*(12), 5552–5576. Available from https://doi.org/10.1039/c3cs60064e.

Elsabahy, M., & Wooley, K. L. (2015). Data mining as a guide for the construction of cross-linked nanoparticles with low immunotoxicity via control of polymer chemistry and supramolecular assembly. *Accounts of Chemical Research, 48*(6), 1620–1630. Available from https://doi.org/10.1021/acs.accounts.5b00066.

Elsabahy, M., & Wooley, K. L. (2018). Reassessment of nanomaterials immunotoxicity. *Nano Today, 20*, 10–12. Available from https://doi.org/10.1016/j.nantod.2018.01.002.

Elsabahy, M., Li, A., Zhang, F., Sultan, D., Liu, Y., & Wooley, K. L. (2013). Differential immunotoxicities of poly(ethylene glycol)- vs. poly(carboxybetaine)-coated nanoparticles. *Journal of Controlled Release, 172*(3), 641–652. Available from https://doi.org/10.1016/j.jconrel.2013.09.010.

Elsabahy, M., Samarajeewa, S., Raymond, J. E., Clark, C., & Wooley, K. L. (2013). Shell-crosslinked knedel-like nanoparticles induce lower immunotoxicity than their non-crosslinked analogs. *Journal of Materials Chemistry B, 1*(39), 5241–5255. Available from https://doi.org/10.1039/c3tb20668h.

Elsabahy, M., Shrestha, R., Clark, C., Taylor, S., Leonard, J., & Wooley, K. L. (2013). Multifunctional hierarchically assembled nanostructures as complex stage-wise dual-delivery systems for coincidental yet differential trafficking of siRNA and paclitaxel. *Nano Letters, 13*(5), 2172–2181. Available from https://doi.org/10.1021/nl4006645.

Elsabahy, M., Wooley, K. L., Hendricksen, A., & Oh, K. (2019). Multiplexing techniques for measurement of the immunomodulatory effects of particulate materials: Precautions when testing micro- and nano-particles. *Methods, 158*, 81–85. Available from https://doi.org/10.1016/j.ymeth.2019.01.006.

Elsabahy, M., Zhang, S., Zhang, F., Deng, Z. J., Lim, Y. H., Wang, H., Parsamian, P., Hammond, P. T., & Wooley, K. L. (2013). Surface charges and shell crosslinks each play significant roles in mediating degradation, biofouling, cytotoxicity and immunotoxicity for polyphosphoester-based nanoparticles. *Scientific Reports, 3*. Available from https://doi.org/10.1038/srep03313.

Greenwood, H. I. (2019). Abbreviated protocol breast MRI: The past, present, and future. *Clinical Imaging, 53*, 169–173. Available from https://doi.org/10.1016/j.clinimag.2018.10.017.

Henriksen, E. L., Carlsen, J. F., Vejborg, I. M. M., Nielsen, M. B., & Lauridsen, C. A. (2019). The efficacy of using computer-aided detection (CAD) for detection of breast cancer in mammography screening: a systematic review. *Acta Radiologica, 60*(1), 13–18. Available from https://doi.org/10.1177/0284185118770917.

Hong, E., & Dobrovolskaia, M. A. (2019). Addressing barriers to effective cancer immunotherapy with nanotechnology: Achievements, challenges, and roadmap to the next generation of nanoimmunotherapeutics. *Advanced Drug Delivery Reviews, 141*, 3–22. Available from https://doi.org/10.1016/j.addr.2018.01.005.

Houdaihed, L., Evans, J. C., & Allen, C. (2017). Overcoming the road blocks: Advancement of block copolymer micelles for cancer therapy in the clinic. *Molecular Pharmaceutics, 14*(8), 2503–2517. Available from https://doi.org/10.1021/acs.molpharmaceut.7b00188.

Ilinskaya, A. N., & Dobrovolskaia, M. A. (2016). Understanding the immunogenicity and antigenicity of nanomaterials: Past, present and future. *Toxicology and Applied Pharmacology, 299*, 70–77. Available from https://doi.org/10.1016/j.taap.2016.01.005.

Jani, D., Allinson, J., Berisha, F., Cowan, K. J., Devanarayan, V., Gleason, C., Jeromin, A., Keller, S., Khan, M. U., Nowatzke, B., Rhyne, P., & Stephen, L. (2016). Recommendations for use and fit-for-purpose validation of biomarker multiplex ligand binding assays in drug development. *AAPS Journal*, *18*(1), 1–14. Available from https://doi.org/10.1208/s12248-015-9820-y.

Kim, B. K., Lee, J. W., Park, P. J., Shin, Y. S., Lee, W. Y., Lee, K. A., Ye, S., Hyun, H., Kang, K. N., Yeo, D., Kim, Y., Ohn, S. Y., Noh, D. Y., & Kim, C. W. (2009). The multiplex bead array approach to identifying serum biomarkers associated with breast cancer. *Breast Cancer Research*, *11*(2). Available from https://doi.org/10.1186/bcr2247.

Ławicki, S., Będkowska, G., Wojtukiewicz, M., & Szmitkowski, M. (2013). Hematopoietic cytokines as tumor markers in breast malignancies. A multivariate analysis with ROC curve in breast cancer patients. *Advances in Medical Sciences*, *58*(2), 207–215. Available from https://doi.org/10.2478/ams-2013-0023.

Leroux, J. C. (2017). Editorial: Drug delivery: Too much complexity, not enough reproducibility? *Angewandte Chemie – International Edition*, *56*(48), 15170–15171. Available from https://doi.org/10.1002/anie.201709002.

Li, L., Chen, L., Zhang, W., Liao, Y., Chen, J., Shi, Y., & Luo, S. (2017). Serum cytokine profile in patients with breast cancer. *Cytokine*, *89*, 173–178. Available from https://doi.org/10.1016/j.cyto.2015.12.017.

Lyon, D., Walter, J., Munro, C. L., Schubert, C. M., & McCain, N. L. (2011). Challenges in interpreting cytokine biomarkers in biobehavioral research: A breast cancer exemplar. *Biological Research for Nursing*, *13*(1), 25–31. Available from https://doi.org/10.1177/1099800410383304.

Ma, C., Nepal, M., Kim, J. H., Fan, P., & Fei, P. (2019). A new look at molecular biology of breast cancer. *Cancer Biology and Therapy*, *20*(1), 1–5. Available from https://doi.org/10.1080/15384047.2018.1507259.

Shrestha, R., Elsabahy, M., Florez-Malaver, S., Samarajeewa, S., & Wooley, K. L. (2012). Endosomal escape and siRNA delivery with cationic shell crosslinked knedel-like nanoparticles with tunable buffering capacities. *Biomaterials*, *33*(33), 8557–8568. Available from https://doi.org/10.1016/j.biomaterials.2012.07.054.

Zhang, F., Elsabahy, M., Zhang, S., Lin, L. Y., Zou, J., & Wooley, K. L. (2013). Shell crosslinked knedel-like nanoparticles for delivery of cisplatin: Effects of crosslinking. *Nanoscale*, *5*(8), 3220–3225. Available from https://doi.org/10.1039/c3nr34320k.

Index

Note: Page numbers followed by "*f*," "*t*," and "*b*" refer to figures, tables, and boxes, respectively.

O

P

Kolibri 360 GmbH
Ferdinand-Jühlke-Straße 7
99095 Erfurt, Deutschland
produktsicherheit@kolibri360.de